Psychosexual Counseling in Andrological Surgery

Elena Vittoria Longhi • Giorgio Franco
Fulvio Colombo

Psychosexual Counseling in Andrological Surgery

A Multidisciplinary Approach to the Patient and His Family

Springer

Elena Vittoria Longhi
Department of Urology Sexual
Medical Center
San Raffaele Hospital
Milano
Italy

Giorgio Franco
Department of Urology
Sapienza University
Rome
Italy

Fulvio Colombo
Andrology Unit
Sant'Orsola University Hospital
Bologna
Italy

ISBN 978-3-319-99644-8   ISBN 978-3-319-99646-2 (eBook)
https://doi.org/10.1007/978-3-319-99646-2

Library of Congress Control Number: 2019930092

This Springer imprint is published by the registered company Springer Nature Switzerland AG
The registered company address is: Gewerbestrasse 11, 6330 Cham, Switzerland

Foreword

The Centre for Sexual Medicine at the Department of Urology, IRCCS San Raffaele, Milan, Italy, was established in 2000. Eighteen years on from the first integrated andrologist-sexologist approach, and under my scientific direction, Prof. Andrea Salonia and Dr. Elena Longhi have adopted a multidisciplinary approach to resolving male and female sexual dysfunctions, of pathological, surgical, and psychogenic origin.

Clinical and research activities have often shown how the andro-sexological approach delves deep into the clinical and interpersonal reasoning of each individual patient.

In this way, a personalized approach toward the patient, the clinical history, and the couple's relationship and toward the implications of the same for the quality of life of each individual is built, thus favoring a strong therapeutic contract and the patient's compliance.

Discussing psychosexological rehabilitation in the andrological surgical approach may seem reductive, but team discussion of each individual surgical theme highlighted in this text offers an analysis of the variants of the pathology and above all an in-depth approach to the individual themes of the patient and the partner.

The surgeon, the psychosexologist, and the medical and paramedical staff constantly interface to promote patient compliance and to accompany the patient from diagnosis to hospitalization, from surgical treatment to discharge, and from the resumption of sexuality to dealing with everyday life.

What kind of psychosexologist are we talking about? A clinician, familiar with the use of video recordings of surgery, an expert in neurological and psychiatric rehabilitation, with training in psychotherapy but no stranger to the clinic. How is this achieved? Not without neuropsychological knowledge of post-traumatic stress and the resulting behavior dynamics.

A hyper-specialized team, respectful of one another's competences and accustomed to debate and communication, where the psychosexologist becomes a "facilitator" of the clinical and therapeutic process, a support for the emotionality of the patient and the partner (or family), and a counsellor for the surgical team, all of these functions are performed with professionalism and empathy.

Each therapeutic team has its own communicative style and a volitive clinical approach, and the choice of the psychosexologist cannot ignore these characteristics.

Francesco Montorsi
Department of Urology
Vita-Salute San Raffaele University
Milan, Italy

Foreword

On the Importance of the Sexological Approach in Andrological Surgery

As stated by Dr. Leonore Tiefer, the ability to procreate, to fulfill the conjugal duty and potency are requirements for the male role everywhere in the world. Before some years, as medical professionals, we still called the loss of this male role "impotence." We have since recognized that "erectile dysfunction" is probably better terminology, for according to Kelley when a man says to his partner that he is impotent, he is saying much more than that his penis cannot become erect. In spite of progressing insights and nuances in the definitions used in the field of andrology, feelings of impotence in the male role as a whole still accompany many andrological conditions such as Peyronie's disease, erectile dysfunction, penile cancer, infertility, and low testosterone. It is evident that throughout the course of these conditions, from the first symptoms to diagnosis to treatment, the sexologist plays an important role in guiding these men by counselling to achieve an increased understanding and acceptance of their condition, as well as defining realistic treatment goals and/or alternative strategies to keep enjoying their sex life.

There are several examples where the sexologist comes in to play a key role in achieving the best attainable result in andrological surgery. The technical and mechanical success of penile implant surgery has been evidenced by a large body of literature. However, thoroughly conducted follow-up studies show that a relatively large proportion of patients and partners fail to achieve sexual satisfaction, and a surprising proportion only infrequently uses their prosthesis. In this setting, both pre- and postoperative (psycho) sexological guidance of the couple has proven successful in both setting realistic expectations, as well as identification of barriers in the postoperative period to resume sex successfully, especially taking into account the fact that these couples have frequently been devoid of penetrative and/or other forms of sexual activity for long periods of time between diagnosing erectile dysfunction and final surgical treatment. They have often undergone a series of unsuccessful and thus frequently disappointing medical approaches, further decreasing their self-confidence. Likewise, sexological counselling may just as well be an integral part in a holistic vision toward incorporation of intracavernosal injections or PDE5 inhibitor therapy in a couple's sex life. In our institute, we do indeed send the large majority of penile implant candidates to the sexologists to receive additional counselling. While the urologist often focusses on the technical aspects of surgery and erectile dysfunction treatment, the sexologist creates realistic expectations on the impact of penile implant surgery on the couple's sexual dynamic.

Peyronie's disease is a currently incurable, sexually debilitating fibrotic disease of the penis that results in penile deformity, coital failure, erectile dysfunction, and significant psychological stress for patients and their partners. It has a devastating impact on mental health, as it was shown that an overwhelming 48% of men with this condition develop a clinically meaningful depression. It is therefore important that these patients not only receive medical information on their condition but are also counselled by a psychosexologist on the potential detrimental effect of their condition on their mental and sexual well-being. In terms of surgery, there are currently no ideal surgical solutions for these patients. Just like the disease itself, the surgical procedures currently widely practiced for the treatment of Peyronie's disease can have devastating impact on the patients' self-confidence, body image, and sexual satisfaction as side effects which include penile shortening (plication procedures), numbness or hypesthesia of the glans and foreskin (procedures with mobilization of the neurovascular bundle), and sometimes loss or impairment of spontaneous and erogenous erectile capacity (including the need for penile implant surgery). Again, it is evident that a completely happy patient and partner can only be achieved if both pre- and postoperative sexological counselling is done in a rigorous fashion.

Penile cancer patients form a complex group of patients who do not only face the fear for the life-threatening aspect of their disease but also undergo often mutilating and disfiguring surgery to treat the primary tumor. While advances in organ-sparing surgery have been made over the past decades, a significant proportion of patients still face penile loss, shortening, or surgeries that—while preserving the erectile capacity—have a lasting impact on the esthetical aspects and sensation of the penis. The fears and worries surrounding both quality and quantity of life issues in this group of patients should be targeted, and regarding the profound impact on sexual function, the psychosexologist is indeed best suited to execute this delicate task.

Summarizing, the role of the psychosexologist in counselling, guiding, and treating patients planned to undergo or having undergone andrological surgical procedures cannot be underestimated and is of capital importance in a modern holistic and patient-centered healthcare setting. In this book, Dr. Longhi and colleagues provide more in-depth and detailed information on the various aspects of psychosexology for andrological surgical patients, which I am sure will help you forward in developing your practice in this field. I wish the reader a pleasant and educative read.

Maarten Albersen
Department of Urology
University Hospitals Leuven
Leuven, Belgium

Foreword

I divided the first years of my medical career between the hospital and my family doctor's practice and I was often confronted with the stories of patients who had to undergo, or had undergone, andrological surgery. At that time, especially for prostate surgery, the arrival of complications such as incontinence and the inability to achieve or maintain an erection were unfortunately frequent. And when one touches the sphere of one's sexuality, while realizing that that intervention had probably saved one's life, the patient's anxiety about the possible consequences is very high. I accompanied several patients to the operating theater and followed them up over time. They told me, sometimes in desperation, of how their sex lives had changed, how their relationship with their partner had changed, and also how their approach to a new woman had changed. Of the fear of "not doing it," despite the arrival of drugs for erectile dysfunction, which worked very well. Of retrograde ejaculation or lack of ejaculation. In short, a different perception of one's body. Of a life marked by before and after the operation. Well then, at that time I really needed to have alongside me a professional such as the author and editor of this book, able to explain how to deal with the possible outcomes of these operations. Someone able to explain that often it is only fear that stops things working, that sensitivity and orgasm can be different, but always pleasant. And that you are men even without the prostate. Also to explain to partners how to deal with a new sexual life as a couple.

Today, with the arrival of "robotic surgery," things have changed. However, patients' concern over this type of intervention remains very great. For this reason, the role of the psychosexologist is—and will remain—essential. To quickly "reactivate" the patient, and help him to resume a sexual life, maybe different, but nonetheless rewarding.

Stefano Vella
National Centre for Global Health,
Higher Institute of Health
Rome, Italy

Foreword

Uro-Oncological Surgery is a delicate surgery, which both in the case of Radical Cystectomy and in the case of Radical Prostatectomy affects the sexual function of our patients.

In recent years, our surgery has undergone an exponential evolution. We have moved from open surgery to laparoscopic surgery and, more recently, to robotic surgery. Already with laparoscopy, the operation had become much less traumatic involving much less physical effort for the patient. In fact, what we call the "surgical disease" was absent. The absence of pain in the postoperative period, the conservation of blood crisis due to the lack of hemorrhaging and, in synthesis, prompt recovery, had an extremely positive impact on the patient. With robotic surgery, this situation has further moved in a positive direction given the greater precision of the operation, which has resulted in even less trauma for the patient.

Moreover, it would be very regrettable if the surgeon were to think of solving all the problems associated with these destructive operations by means of surgery alone.

A destructive act by definition but one that today, thanks to the increase in our knowledge and the synergy with psychology, sexology, and neuro-urology, enables us to see the patient not as the bearer of a life-threatening disease but as a person who can and must be helped in a positive way in his journey toward a "Restitutio ad integrum."

In 1999, I did an epistolary survey of about 500 patients who underwent radical prostatectomy and, to my surprise, many of them complained that they had not received adequate psychological or functional support after surgery. This last word comprised not only the rehabilitation phase of continence but also the resumption of sexual activity. It was obvious to me that the surgeon does not have the ability, the training, or even the time to follow his patients through this rehabilitation process. It was then that I realized the need to organize a team of professionals to fill this void.

The first aspect, perhaps the most important, was undoubtedly the psychosexual aspect. In fact, neuro-urological rehabilitation is able to accelerate the recovery of urinary continence, but it is the loss of sexual life that can easily lead the patient to a quite severe depression.

In our shared work experience, we have learned many things that you will find in the framework of this valuable book. I would also like to draw your attention to the importance of a patient–psychologist relationship that must begin even before the surgical operation and precisely within that limbo that leads from diagnosis, with its surgical indication, to the moment of hospitalization.

Those are the days, and unfortunately sometimes weeks, in which the patient is abandoned to himself and accumulates sometimes deadly amounts of stress. All this can be avoided or at least corrected, with appropriate and professional psychological assistance.

The other very important phase is obviously the postoperative rehabilitation phase, where the collaboration between the psychologist and the patient should always be extended to the partner as well. In fact, a therapy without the involvement of the partner would have little chance of success and in our experience we have seen that the best results are obtained when the couple functions well.

I would like to close these few words with a heartfelt thanks to Dr. Elena Longhi who has helped us in recent years to become aware of our patients' problems. The multidisciplinary approach to postoperative rehabilitation has certainly helped our patients, but it has also enabled us surgeons to better perform our profession.

Vito Pansadoro
Department of Urology
Pio XI Hospital
Rome, Italy

Preface

There are many ways to practice a profession as delicate and complex as that of the psychosexologist. I have always chosen to learn: from doctors, surgeons, nurses, and patients. I was fortunate to have many mentors who gave me the opportunity to enter the operating theater, to understand the complexity of their profession, to learn their language. Practical, certain, and capable of turning all sorts of knowledge into action. Without hierarchy and without competition.

I was welcomed by the most experienced nurses, not only so that I might learn about pharmacological formulations but above all about the ways of administering them, not without space for communication but listening to the patient and family members.

Although coming from a background in psychological studies, I studied these disciplines on the ward, transforming my profession into that of a clinician who learns rather than remaining in the realms of a science which, due to prejudice, is often perceived as "vague, made of abstract words, of emptiness."

While specializing, I was fascinated by the publication by Milton Erickson, entitled *My Voice Will Go with You*.

I have personally experienced, speaking with patients, during these years as a professional, that very often I have become, against my will, a mental ritual for many of them: "I was reminded of what you told me Doctor and ..." "I did my homework, like you told me to ..." "how many times you came to mind ...."

I feel lucky to have always had patients motivated to tell me their story, their knowledge of life, sharing with me the deepest part of their sensitivity. They have taught me to have a "centimeter more of courage than of fear" and to want to build at any cost. Maybe I also projected a part of my personal history. I owe my survival to a neonatal surgeon.

Since then, I have always tried to see beyond the pathology, to make the patient as much a protagonist in the disease as in health.

This book, the first of a trilogy, on Clinical Sexuality aims to show how the multidisciplinary approach satisfies all the protagonists. Among the specialists, it facilitates communication, intensifying interpersonal and professional relations without affecting their clinical autonomy or their contract of trust with the patient. I still think that the contract par excellence is between the andrologist surgeon and the patient, while the psychosexologist is a "facilitator of the entire therapeutic process of the individual patient."

As I often say, "a bespoke tailor" invests in the individual patient and not in the pathology, making a unique approach, not forgetting the discussion with doctors, surgeons, and nurses.

The stories of patients and their partners show how the process of the disease also highlights "the couple's contract," the type of relationship between the two, the sexuality, the plans for the future, the relationship with physicality, and the relationship with the medical environment and hospitalization.

Even patients who are "difficult" in character or temperament are often the "supervisors of a medical team" which sometimes gets distracted, gets too involved, and has difficulty communicating with any type of patient. Even doctors, like the rest of humanity, sometimes struggle to communicate with characters removed from their own sensitivity, and the psychosexologist may be helpful in easing tensions, misunderstandings, or just fear or fatigue reactions, on both sides.

The psychosexologist: a deus ex machina? Certainly not. Rather, a clinician who wants to make every meeting with a colleague, a patient, and a family member a motive for learning and well-being.

It is customary to thank the experts in these cases and to give them heartfelt gratitude. I like to turn my gratitude to anyone, doctor, patient, family member, who has allowed me to enter their life and motivate a new narrative.

I thank the one who taught me to respect the fragilities of others, to stimulate healthy female enterprise, and never to be without a smile, a feeling, and a human and therapeutic complicity, with humor and simplicity: my father.

Milan, Italy Elena Vittoria Longhi

Preface

Cooperating with a Psycho-sexologist in Surgical Andrology—The Andrologist's Perspective

Compared to other surgical fields, andrological surgery entails specific psychological aspects and peculiarities. In any kind of surgery, in fact, patient expectations and hopes are usually very high since it is considered the faster and more effective solution in resolving the problem in a definitive way. However, when the problem entails his sexual organs, the penis in particular, and his sexuality, psychological implications are usually deeper and more consistent and therefore expectations are even higher. Body images, concerns, and dysmorphophobias are also magnified and are of relevance when dealing with the genitals compared to other body parts. This is why when we assess an andrological patient and offer him a surgical solution, a special care has to be given to the immediate and delayed psychological consequences of that procedure on that specific patient. Although in some instances the sensitivity and experience of the urologist–andrologist might be enough to evaluate and address the psychosexual aspects of a patient to be operated on, in most situations the help of a psycho-sexologist is advisable.

For example, patients who develop penile deformities due to fibrous plaques of Peyronie's disease are commonly psychologically distressed for the deformity and indications to surgery must be properly addressed by the andrologist after careful assessment of their psychological status and real reason for distress: penile aesthetic appearance, difficulties or discomfort during intercourse, dyspareunia, presence of erectile dysfunction. Indications to and type of surgical reconstruction may vary significantly according to the reason of distress perceived by the patient. Another typical situation is represented by the youngster who requests augmentative surgery for a supposed inadequate size of his genitalia (dysmorphophobia), or by the old patient who requires a penile hydraulic prosthesis implantation. The psychological implications of all these conditions are often better detected and investigated by a dedicated psycho-sexologist, with a structured interview or with the aid of specific questionnaires aiming at assessing the impact of the condition on the patient well-being, mood and sexual life, and the chances of surgery to improve patient satisfaction and psychological status [1, 2].

Therefore, there are many reasons why a psychological consultation represents an advantage, if not a necessity, in the assessment and treatment of andrological patients who require a surgical procedure.

And what about the drawbacks of patient referral to a psycho-sexologist? Probably the only ones are represented by increased costs and time, or by the patient refusal of a psychological assistance not to be considered a "psychological patient." To partly avoid this last situation, an optimal care might be represented by a combined simultaneous patient consultation by the andrologist and the psychologist, but this situation is hardly possible and logistically difficult. What appears to be a good solution is to refer patients to the psychologist specifically trained in sexology, providing specific questions or surgical indications, maybe grouping them on specific days in the same consultation room of the andrologist. Patient will be happy to be thoroughly investigated preoperatively in the same center without feeling himself a "psychological patient." The andrologist will take his final decision after reviewing the psychologic consultation report.

Once the indication to surgery has been confirmed, special attention is to be made to the informed consent acquisition. Legal considerations are in fact very important in this kind of surgery. Experience has shown that in andrological surgery the rate of legal litigation is higher than other kind of surgery. First of all, an accurate psychosexual history and physical examination must be obtained. After this, a careful explanation of the proposed intervention, and of its most frequent complications, has to be given, possibly with the aid of drawings and schemes. The psychologist in many instances can help the patient in the understanding and decision-making process of giving the consent to surgery.

In conclusion, when dealing with surgery and its consequences, psycho-sexologists are the andrologists' best friends!

Rome, Italy — G. Franco
Bologna, Italy — F. Colombo

References

1. Spyropoulos E, Galanakis I, Dellis A (2007) Augmentation phalloplasty patient selection and satisfaction inventory: a novel questionnaire to evaluate patients considered for augmentation phalloplasty surgery because of penile dysmorphophobia. Urology 70(2)
2. Schieber K, Kollei I, De Zwaan M, Martin A et al (2015) Classification of body dysmorphic disorder—what is the advantage of the new DSM-5 criteria? J Psychosom Res 78:223–227

Contents

Contributors

Fulvio Colombo Head of the Andrology Unit, Sant'Orsola University Hospital, Bologna, Italy

Fabio Ferro Consultant Expert in Genital Surgery, Department of Surgery, Bambino Gesù Children's Hospital, Research Institute, Rome, Italy

Alessandro Franceschelli Head of the Andrology Unit, "S.Orsola" University Hospital, Bologna, Italy

Francesco Franceschelli Head of the Andrology Unit, "S.Orsola" University Hospital, Bologna, Italy

Giorgio Franco Department of Gynaecological and Urological Sciences, Sapienza University of Rome, Rome, Italy

Elena Vittoria Longhi Department of Urology, Sexual Medical Center, IRCCS San Raphael Hospital, Vita and Salute University, Milan, Italy

Paolo Maria Michetti Dipartimento di Scienze Ginecologico-Ostetriche, E Scienze Urologiche—Università La Sapienza, Roma, Italy

Leonardo Misuraca "Regina Elena" National Cancer Institute, Rome, Italy

Armin Pycha Department of Urology, Central Hospital of Bolzano, Bolzano, Italy

Vito Pansadoro, MD, FRCS (Hon) Department of Urology, Pio XI Hospital, Rome, Italy

Mauro Silvani ASL BI of Biella, Biella, Italy

Emanuela Trenti Department of Urology, Central Hospital of Bolzano, Bolzano, Italy

Part I

Basic Considerations

1 Who Is the Surgical Patient?

1.1 Who Is the Surgical Patient?

Surgical stress certainly does raise fears: fears concerning death, fear of losing control of one's own body, fear of anesthesia, fear of the surgery itself, and the fear of pain after surgery.

Age, sensitivity, character, and the role within the family system are other variables of the adolescent and/or adult, which may affect the surgical path. This is especially true when considering the family as a whole. Not only the patient but also the wider family too is affected by the diagnosis. However, if we consider the "family body," it is as if the whole unit is lying down on the operating table.

The fear of losing the familiar and the anguish of postsurgical complications cause family roles to be expressed with anxiety and irritability. Requests for reassurance from the surgeon and the search for information on the internet are just two aspects of the anguish of separation.

For a teenager to undergo surgery inevitably leads the family to speculate about their loss and the anguish of a future without meaning. This perspective increases the apprehension or even the certainty of the failure to overcome the event, leading to states of anguish, passivity, helplessness, mistrust and the idea of the worthlessness of their endeavors.

Thus, just as with the person nominated for surgery, the feeling of not being in a position to manage their own lives, and of being at the mercy of uncontrollable events, increases.

For this reason, giving the correct information step by step is fundamental. Doctor-patient-family communication builds a trust agreement with the surgeon, while the patient's postsurgical compliance builds an alliance between medical and paramedical staff and the family. A clinical path is shared by the doctors and the unknowing therapists (the family and the patient).

Although making the diagnosis is of course in the surgeon's competence, the patient and family members also have their own diagnoses. "I felt pain for months but I was scared...." "We should have made more frequent checks ...," "Why did it

E. V. Longhi et al., *Psychosexual Counseling in Andrological Surgery*,
https://doi.org/10.1007/978-3-319-99646-2_1

have to happen to us?" These remain largely silent thoughts but are a source of doubt, suspicion, and distrust of the doctor's reassurances.

What to do? It's not about forcing the patient to talk about himself but rather about being ready to listen to him and to give him an opportunity to express his views.

Leading by the hand along the path ahead: the specialist's consultations (anesthesiologist), the importance of fasting from midnight (to prevent aspiration pneumonia), rest prior to surgery, the chances of any blood transfusions (reassurance about blood born infections and the possibility of auto transfusion), explanations of the reasons for trichotomy (to decrease the risk of skin infection, the usual host of bacteria), and the postoperative use of painkillers.

Research has made it clear that accurate information about all of these points has a positive impact on the operating course: reduces the length of hospital stays and the use of analgesics and minimizes the fear of the postoperative path and of being discharged.

But that is not all.

From the time of diagnosis, the patient enters a post-traumatic process that will last on average for 90–120 days. The body increases the release of acetylcholine (ombudsman of the nerve impulse), corticosteroids (to maintain adequate circulatory volume), catecholamines, and certain hormonal substances that control energy production in the vital organs.

Also the body generally produces a larger amount of the stress hormone cortisol, which however causes poor control over emotions. Sharing this information with the patient means de-pathologizing his anguish and rehabilitating him in a clinical process of which he has hitherto been unaware, which is also the cause of frustration, loss of control, and fear of making plans.

Preoperative anxiety can provoke aggressive reactions, an increase in distress and a deterioration in the quality of life of the patient. Pain management may be more difficult in the postoperative stage, and higher doses of anesthetic may be required during surgery, while there may also be lower satisfaction with the treatment.

Insecurity, restlessness, depression, insomnia, muscle tension, and nightmares can often be traced to the passivity of the hospitalized patient, leading to a feeling of dependence on medical and paramedical staff.

Scrutiny of these disorders is fundamental when deciding which preventive interventions are necessary during the preoperative phase, in order to exclude minor psychiatric disorders.

It is important to note that these disorders affect a high percentage of patients who flock to specialized health services but are then not diagnosed.

Many studies have shown a higher prevalence of depression in surgical patients than in the general population [1]. Thus, a correlation between preoperative anxiety (state of anxiety) and trait anxiety levels linked to the personality of the patient has been found.

The presence of pain, intense or moderate, increases the risk of preoperative anxiety, as does the type of surgery and its psychological impact on the patient. It is no coincidence that many patients recall interventions of circumcision or of varicocele in adolescence as indelible traumas, causing poor penile sensitivity in adulthood.

Patients who smoke have a higher risk of developing anxiety before the intervention because they develop withdrawal symptoms during hospitalization. Previous experience of small surgical intervention though reduces the risk of preoperative anxiety.

The opportunity to undergo an intervention under "day surgery" is one factor that studies have shown to be a lesser cause of preoperative anxiety: the thought that it will all end in one day and that the patient can return home in the afternoon and sleep in his own bed make the wait for the operation less insidious [2].

1.2 How Much Influence Is the Hospital Setting?

The hospital is by its nature an environment dedicated to curing. Once admitted, individuals cease to be people and become patients.

From a medical and surgical perspective, they become individuals in need of diagnosis, hospitalization, treatment, surgery, prognosis, and follow-up. For the person and the family, this means entering a context where their power of control and of sharing the care depends on the underlying disease, the diagnosis of the surgeon, and the prospect of healing proposed by him.

In practice, they depend on the surgeon and the hospital team. None or few consider the distress of the family: the hospital is, for them, often a cause of frustration and insecurity.

This begins with the lack of living space and autonomy in the patient's room, as well as the difficulty in understanding thoroughly the diagnostic and therapeutic terms of the doctors and nurses.

Often I read in their eyes, "will the situation be bad?" "What if it doesn't go well? What will be the future of the younger… or the adult ...?"

Anxiety is very common and aggression is a response to fear and dissatisfaction: nurses appear to be in a hurry, and the surgeon seems too quick to give clinical explanations and to reassure the family.

This at least is the feeling of many family members and some patients: "Doctor, I'm in a lot of pain." And the surgeon replied, "It's perfectly normal, don't worry."

The patient and the family cannot be comforted. Even a few days in hospital involves depression, isolation, a sense of regression, concerns about the post, stress about impotence, and inadequacy in the face of the patient's suffering.

And then? What about the andrological diagnosis? Whenever a teenager undergoes surgery to the genital region, the apprehension of the parents becomes progressive. Involuntarily, the mothers blame themselves for not having been able to deliver a healthy child. The fathers, in turn, feel responsible and concerned about not being adequate masculine role models.

Then, other silent doubts of the parents are as follows: "will this boy be a normal man?" "Will he want a woman like all his peers?" "Will he have an adequate body like all the other boys?"

To whom should these concerns be addressed? Often they are filtered through requests to the surgeon for reassurance, "will everything be OK afterwards?," or continuous searches for information, more or less plausible, through the Internet, to understand something more and to avert the worst.

The attitudes of many parents toward nurses and doctors, seemingly anxious, aggressive, and nagging, are only cries for comfort to quell the anxiety of "losing forever" the hospitalized boy or adult.

There is nothing like surgery to raise the specter of loss and death. Even for a varicocele? It sounds crazy, but that's the way it is.

It is not the diagnosis that brings out these anxieties, varicocele, circumcision, etc. They are evoked simply by the fear of not being able to control one's life.

This is the anguish of not being able to make plans for the future, of losing the freedom to live according to one's own wishes. It is the anesthesia, the hospitalization, and the surgery that invade with a scalpel the genital area of a boy or an adult that influences the thoughts and behavior of the patient and the family.

It is the surgery that disrupts the manly feelings of both the young man and the experienced adult. Emotionally surgery is often seen as an inevitable intrusion, but not hard to deal with a bit of courage.

1.3 What Does the Surgeon See?

The relationship between the surgeon and the andrological surgical patient is complex: on the one hand, there is the specialist, responsible for the health of the patient both clinically and legally.

On the other there is an individual who puts himself totally in the surgeon's hands. At best, it is a relationship of trust and dependency for the patient. For the surgeon, it is a human clinical contract for which he assumes all responsibility.

Being aware that intervention could also have unwanted outcomes or might not succeed, with whom do they share their anxieties? It could be argued that they are part of the chosen profession. Certainly, but over time, clinical experience enhances increasingly sophisticated surgical techniques and applications.

At the same time, the sensitivity of the surgeon makes him/her increasingly aware of not being able to cope with the anxiety of the patient, because he himself/she herself is charged with responsibilities and anguish.

Therefore the surgeon can only control his/her own anxieties and leave those of the patient and family to the psychosexologist.

1.4 The Psychosexologist's Role

The psychosexologist is a surgeon's ally and loyal partner, who gives only practical information to enhance the doctor-patient partnership and reassure the family.

One who appears alongside him, in the best case scenario, is right there from the first andrological visit. A clinical partnership for one patient and one family, two specialists, is accustomed to working side by side, giving answers beyond diagnosis.

In everyday life it is more common for the psychosexologist to be introduced to the patient and family at the second meeting, once the surgical route has been outlined.

Why? The psychosexologist is generally a facilitator of the surgical process at this early stage.

As already outlined, he/she describes, in empathetic terms, the clinical treatment already outlined by the surgeon:

Pleased to meet you. I know it's not an easy time for you. For this reason the surgeon wants you to be accompanied on this path and not to feel alone. Is everything clear? What are your thoughts after the first visit with the surgeon?

The surgeon and the psychosexologist are a pairing with distinct therapeutic roles: the surgeon organizes the surgical treatment in detail with the operating team and hospital staff.

The psychosexologist calls for a further meeting with the teenager to get a picture of his acquired sexual education, his fears resulting from the diagnosis, parental expectations about his prognosis, and, usually, his school and sporting life and his friends.

Relations with any siblings or the condition of an only child are also considered.

For verification, the psychosexologist also meets the parents of the teenager with the patient present:

Are you concerned about your parents?
Who do you think is more concerned?

Hence the psychosexologist tries to get a picture of the family roles, the figure that supports the clan and how, emotionally, the teenager feels he might disappoint the family if he does not become the man that mum and dad would like, even in the sphere of health and sexuality.

What is it all for? In clinical terms, it is to be able to inform the surgeon about the communicative style to adopt with the family, how to positively influence the patient's compliance and to hypothesize anxiolytic or antidepressant therapy for the patient during the hospital stay, and whether the adolescent is emotionally fragile.

What more?

As Schneider reports (1969), the surgeon cannot identify with the sick, because otherwise he/she could not carry out most of his/her duties.

The surgeon cannot be carried away by the emotional nature of the patient, whether adolescent or adult, but must understand the individual on a human level, identifying, with the help of the psychosexologist, a suitable therapy, that is, the degree of cooperation and positive responsiveness of the patient to surgery, the prognosis, and the resumption of daily activities.

The psychosexologist is therefore present on the ward, talking to the nurses, the patient, and family members, concerning himself/herself with the emotional responses and the resilience of each of them.

He/she consults with the surgeon and proposes, subsequent to discharge, a meeting with the patient to share any emotional reactions resulting from postsurgical stress and the subsequent recovery of sexuality.

Unlike the therapeutic contract with the surgeon, the collaboration between psychosexologist and patient is short term.

While the surgeon can follow the patient from the check-ups to prevention visits and can become a lifelong reference point, the psychosexologist must remove him/herself from the lives of the patient and family members.

In doing so, the psychosexologist delivers into the hands of the patient a fitting masculinity able to be experienced autonomously, without further intrusion.

What about the psychosexologist? Are we not led to believe that each time the psychosexologist has completed his/her personalized projects, he/she feels, like all humans, a moment of abandonment and loneliness? He/she has been trained for short-term clinical relationships and is expected to be the first to abandon and live as part of a medical team sharing countless stories, stories of families, partners, nurses, doctors, and nonmedical personnel, apart from their own, silently, side by side with everyone, without complaint.

1.5 Conclusion

Andrological surgery requires a clinical approach. Each patient, adolescent or adult, faces andrological diagnosis at a time in life when surgery hasn't been planned.

As a result, the patient alternates between feelings of anxiety and the anguish of losing control of his life, as do family members.

The surgical medical team and the psychosexologist inevitably become a reference for health and the continuity of life. From them, understanding, respect, dedication, and professionalism are required.

The harmony between the medical and paramedical staff and the figure of the psychosexologist appears to be an important prerequisite for the patient and the family. The more closely the reference team communicates and interfaces, the more the patient and family feel engaged in a continuing health process.

The patient's sexuality, be he adolescent or adult, is not only a physiological response. It becomes an expression of his role in the world, of his power to control his own actions, and of his confidence to compete with others, to be desirable to the female world.

The nonsexual aspects of andrological surgery underlie the ability of the individual to feel secure in his relationship with the world, deserving of the affections of a woman.

Understanding everything and sharing as a team means treating the patient as "a single individual," avoiding psychological complications to surgery, removing any element of discomfort or dissatisfaction on the part of the patient in relation to surgical treatment right from the start.

References

1. Vaeroy H (2003) Prevalence of depression among general hospital surgical inpatients. Nordic J Psychiatric LVII(1):13–16
2. James D (2000) Patient perceptions of day surgery. Br J Perioper Nurs X(9):262–269

2 Illness and Individual Reactions

The occurrence of disease is not without consequences on the psychological status of families of surgical patients. They often need outside help to communicate, react, understand and cope with the new situation and the destabilization caused by the disease.

The patient and his family experience, before and after surgery, a sense of worthlessness. During hospitalization they must give up school and professional activity, their homes, routines, long-standing appointments, trips, night outs, the gym, and friends from dance class.

The disease and the hospitalization become a snag, an obstacle to the realization of projects in progress and to professional, scholastic, economic, and social satisfaction.

Into all of this fit the patient's individuality and the character of each family member. The same diagnosis and the same surgical path may occasionally have several different reactions on the part of the patient and of the family members who support him.

These variables are used to inform the communication style of the surgeon and the clinical team.

2.1 The Four Most Common Communication Styles

The four most common communication styles have been identified as follows:

1. Emotional dependence
2. Emotional counter-dependence
3. Displaced conflict
4. Interdependence

E. V. Longhi et al., *Psychosexual Counseling in Andrological Surgery*,
https://doi.org/10.1007/978-3-319-99646-2_2

2.1.1 Emotional Dependence

The surgeon has a dominant and protective role, reassuring the patient and assuming full emotional and professional responsibility for the diagnosis and the surgery.

The patient and his family assign to the surgeon all responsibility and thus require protection and reassurance.

The surgeon takes on a protective parental role, and patient compliance will be minimal as he behaves like a dependent patient/child, afraid of everything, anxious, hypercritical, and with a low pain threshold.

2.1.2 Emotional Counter-Dependence

The patient and his family assume a hypercritical role toward the surgeon and the clinical team. They show distrust of medical evidence and express a disparaging attitude.

Faced with this challenge, the surgeon exhibits the same critical behavior toward the patient and the family, or, if the surgeon personalizes the relationship, he or she is contrary and strongly critical. Patient compliance in these cases will be much lower than the clinician's expectations, and at every opportunity the family will show dissatisfaction with the care and the surgical technique and with the professional adequacy of the paramedics.

The rehabilitation phase after surgery can only repeat the same patterns: the patient is dissatisfied with the aesthetics of the penis, for example, complains of lack of penile sensitivity, or asks for consultation with more doctors after the surgery in the hope at least one of them will agree with his opinion.

This type of patient shows a pessimistic view of the diagnosis. It is therefore extremely difficult to motivate him properly and to counter preoperative anxiety, fear, and anguish.

In addition, the patient tries to forget the diagnosed disease and, in revenge against the surgeon and himself, takes on behaviors and lifestyles which run counter to the recommendation of the clinician: he leads a sedentary life (instead of practicing a sport), follows a disordered diet, smokes, and does not disdain soft drugs.

2.1.3 Displaced Conflict

This model is characterized by an excess of rationality. The surgeon, the patient, and his family members prefer to deal with the disease only from a technical point of view.

Such patients may appear obsessive in their requests for information from the surgeon, searching the Internet for other opinions, from the perspective of a very scientific doctor-patient relationship.

Needless to say, patient compliance will be proportional to how accommodating the surgeon is in his response. He will demonstrate much rigor and professionalism.

All true? Not quite. These patients are often dishonest when answering the surgeon's questions often responding with half-truths. They only partially follow the advice given and are quick to adopt an ambivalent attitude toward the healthcare professional.

2.1.4 Interdependence

This style is characterized through a mature relationship shared between the surgeon, the patient, and the family, where they agree on a clinical protocol that provides for separate but individual responsibility, concluding with a contract of trust and collaboration also on an empathetic and emotional level.

This certainly appears to be the most mature model, securing patient compliance, the practical and emotional support of the family, and recognition of and gratitude to the medical staff and the surgeon.

Patients who adhere to this model appear curious and interested in managing their own bodies, treating the disease as a mere hiccup, to be dealt with competently and consistently.

They are open to both traditional pharmacology and alternative medicine: they do not easily allow themselves to be influenced by other specialists who do not belong to the clinical staff.

They will also, if required, make lifestyle changes: the heavy smoker continues to smoke but gradually reduces the number of cigarettes. The inactive teenager comes to view sport as a useful tool for health, without feeling himself deprived of hours in front of the computer or in front of the TV.

2.2 Why Did This Happen to Me?

Clinical experience shows that all patients ask the same question "Why did it happen to me?". Starting from this question, the patient recounts his medical history, habits, and lifestyle choices and often concludes "I didn't deserve this."

These patient's "stories" have been identified by Frank [1] as constituting three different types:

1. Stories of restitution
2. Stories of chaos
3. Search stories

2.2.1 Stories of Restitution

These are optimistic stories, aimed at regaining control over the disease ("the enemy"), while surgery, the foolproof weapon, will defeat the diagnosis and normality will return.

This attitude, closer to Western culture, leads us to experience the disease as an entity which is foreign to the patient and family. Also in the language of the patient:

"... this disease has been a bomb ... "

"all my securities have melted like snow in the sun ..."

"I was already worried about the university exams and now (with diagnosis) it never rains but it pours ... "

2.2.2 Stories of Chaos

These stories, unlike the previous two, are dramatic and with no way out. The patient and the family often think that a real recovery will not come about.

The sudden lack of control over their lives drives these patients into chaos: the disease will result in economic problems; it will distract from relationships with girls, and there will be problems with sexuality.

" ... I have never been to hospital..."

"It seemed like a nightmare"

"My life is over at 50. Do you understand? I won't be the man I was before"

2.2.3 Search Stories

These are almost psychological and/or moral stories, in which the disease is seen as a chance to give new meaning to life.

" ... nothing happens by chance ... so that means I have to review my role in the family, my profession, take stock of my life ... "

Attention to healing becomes secondary to the hypothesis of the changes that the disease imposes, so much so that the emotional climate of these stories is even more quiet and peaceful compared to other types, almost a Zen fable.

2.3 Each Patient Has His Waterloo

In addition to what research tells us, day-to-day clinical experience shows us that some patients view disease as a defeat, as in the case of surgical intervention or a course of radiotherapy. Owning a body that is perceived as abnormal affects the sense of male identity, of self-esteem, and of the sexual role.

The aesthetic aspect is undoubtedly an important factor: but what of health and pleasure?

Our real body and the image that each of us has within ourselves are the elements with which we communicate: we know people, we build links, and we experience sexuality.

These functions in a "body violated by surgery" harm self-esteem, the power and the safety to seduce and to be seduced and to love and to be loved. A sick body is perceived by the patient as different, foreign.

But is it possible to say all of this to the surgeon?

It is, especially if the clinician has the humility to avail him/herself of the aid of a psychsexologist who, much more than he/she, possesses the tools to understand the feelings of the patient.

Following the many misunderstandings between surgeon and psychosexologist in my clinical practice, the surgeons and I today share the following approach:

The surgeon to the patient:

... now that we shave agreed the stages of surgery, I would be grateful if you would meet my colleague (psychosexologist) as this will help me to better understand how to help you (the patient) and help (family members: parents in the case of an adolescent, the partner in the case of an adult patient)...respecting your sensitivity

The psychosexologist to the patient:

...How do you think we can help the surgeon? Let him know a little more? What do you make of the situation? What are your most recurring thoughts? What do you think about the surgery?

2.4 From a Small Waterloo to Taking Charge

In this way, the psychosexologist begins to bring out the patient's history, the type of approach to the disease, and the therapeutic compliance expected by the surgeon and the clinical staff.

The teenager's family often reports that they can finally talk about their real problems.

Case History
Stephen, 16 years, needs type II varicocele surgery. The mother admits to being unnerved by the surgery, because Stephen was adopted and has already suffered too much trauma. The father nods and adds "my wife has quit her job to care for Stephen, because he has always been a difficult character." Stephen attends college, doesn't know "what he wants to do when he grows up," and believes that "this disease" is confirmation that the birth mother was right to abandon him: "I'm worthless and now I'm going to disappoint my adoptive parents."

2.4.1 What to Report to the Surgeon?

For example, Stephen is a patient in need of support regarding his capacity to deal with surgery, since he is inclined to depression and self-destructive behavior. In this case an emotional and supportive empathetic style of communication is preferred.

He might have a low pain threshold and disturbed sleep in the postoperative phase due to anxiety about the disease and an anxio-depressive syndrome linked to the difference in his body and him being adopted.

And there's more. Parents often have trouble speaking of disease not only with the sick child but also with their other children, the siblings of the patient.

The reason for this is a desire not to involve them too much in a situation which is for them (the parents) already stressful. There is also the desire not to negatively affect their welfare.

Moreover, failure to apprise the siblings of the conditions of the hospitalized child can arouse in them feelings of jealousy and conflict, due to the excess of care for the patient, to their detriment.

Whereas talking openly about the disease, without dramatizing and with positive emphasis means informing him about the situation in a neutral collaborative way.

Your brother is lucky to have so much support in the family.

This encourages the siblings to live the event as an experience in which each of them can feel useful, important, and necessary: a real team at the side of the medical team.

There's more. Talking to the siblings brings out the degree of perceived risk from a teenager.

Will I get sick too? Is my brother's disease infectious?.

Parents and teenagers with regard to their perception of their own vulnerability to the disease were studied. It turns out that teenagers are less optimistic than adults with respect to the consequences of a lack of attention to health.

It follows then that the psychosexologist in andrological surgery should have a multidisciplinary preparation. He/she must acquired, through clinical experience, research, and a broadening of study, a set of skills, neurological and neuropsychiatric, rehabilitative, pharmacological, surgical (watching videos of interventions), and rehabilitation, in addition to specializations in systemic therapy, sexology, and, in my case, psycho-oncology.

He/she is a multipurpose specialist who works alongside the surgeon to facilitate the patient's clinical process and to adapt the communication between clinicians and paramedics, clinicians and patient, and family and patient, to filter the feelings of conflict, panic, stress, or mere professional tension.

An observer who describes more than one human reality and always tries to find more virtuous connections so that the patient can rediscover his identity, even in sickness and pain.

Psychological factors in postoperative pain control and management are very important. Zoppi [2] identified four aspects in the hospital experience of pain:

1. The patient's historical experience of pain
2. Current control pain
3. Expectation of pain
4. Emotional state

If the prior experience of the patient is immutable, so are the other three dimensions.

Anxiety, depression, and fear amplify the perception of pain by increasing the effect of the algogenic neurotransmitters of the central nervous system and the analgesic effect of depressing neurotransmitters (norepinephrine, serotonin, endorphins).

The interview with the psychosexologist, in the preoperative stage, also assumes this role. Sharing the preparatory steps for surgery, the phase of anesthesia, and accompanying the patient to the preoperative room all describe a process of clinical and emotional collaboration in the field, reducing stress, anxiety, and concern.

2.5 How Should the Psychosexologist Speak?

In no small way, the psychosexologist's manner and style of communication are useful tools in the relationship with both the surgeon and the nursing staff and the patient and the family.

The use of words is equally important, in the preoperative room:

> *... soon you will have a nice sleep and I'm certain that the surgeon, with all his skill, will help you. You are not alone*

In one experience in the United States, a few years ago, the medical team welcomed the patient back from sleep with a round of applause. "When is the operation?," asked the patient. "All done," replied the surgeon, and every member of the team shook his hand, saying "Congratulations!"

Not all cultures accept such theatricality in these circumstances, but there is no doubt that the use of such terminology has great therapeutic value. This positive connotation, for example, helps the medical team and the patient to experience surgical stress at a time of crisis (from the Greek "crisis," meaning the turning point of a disease). A transition from one state of health to another, a "pouring of old wine into new barrels", a constant transition between disease, prevention, health and wellness. In a circular process.

2.6 Disease Is a Citizen of the World

For some patients, the transition from one state of the disease to another appears more complex. Every industrialized country is host to a multiethnic population. According to the World Health Organization (WHO), the right to treatment is essential, and Jirojwong and Manderson [3] have tracked a number of variables that characterize "ethnic" patients:

1. Culture
2. Acculturation
3. The concept of time
4. Linguistic understanding

2.6.1 Culture

The perception of disease and the symptoms that distinguish it can vary from culture to culture, especially when it comes to the genital sphere.

For some cultures, the pelvic region is impure, and this assumption might affect the patient's adaptation to reality and compromise patient compliance to surgical treatment.

If we look at the opposite sex, we encounter the request by mothers in Central Africa to take home the placenta which, when dried, can be ingested together with water or food to profit from its curative properties.

2.6.2 Acculturation

The level of assimilation may make it difficult for the patient to respect his ethnic culture within the host culture. Much will depend on his integration into the host society and the socioeconomic class to which he belongs.

2.6.3 The Concept of Time

It is common for patients of different ethnicities, especially those not fully integrated, to have a very flexible concept of chronological time. They may not respect clinical appointment times and may autonomously vary the timing and methods of taking medical therapies.

The difficulty of explaining to a diabetic patient the need to monitor blood sugar levels daily has been pointed out.

2.6.4 Linguistic Understanding

The healing process can be affected by the poor linguistic competence of ethnically diverse patients when expressing feelings, sensations, and symptoms, as can collaboration in the diagnostic process and following medical recommendations for the pre- and postoperative stages.

2.7 Dealing with Ethnically Diverse Patients

Forming relationships with these patients is not easy, and neither is avoiding prejudices relating to ethnicity, appearance, and communication difficulties.

Even the medical and paramedical staff sometimes find themselves in difficulty, unconsciously assuming an authoritarian attitude that could be perceived as a lack of helpfulness and collaboration.

Hence the use of a technical language in the communication of the diagnosis and surgical methods. Also, it is not unusual for ethnically diverse patients to have a professional qualification or a degree from the country of origin, which is not recognized in the host country. This leads to a factor of greater stress for the individual, who expects a medical reception equal to his social standing.

Moving on to family traditions, some ethnically diverse patients present themselves at visits with several family members or require that the head of the family be present at every hospital procedure. Either they feel limited by religious practices or in the dictates that these determine regarding their relationship with their bodies during the clinical path.

2.8 Conclusions

All these variables, if properly looked into and valued, are part of the surgical process and its success. The value of psychosexologist lies also in bringing out the differences, complicity, and cultural distances in an "individualized project" of accompanying the patient and the family and, above all, in the preoperative stage.

In the postoperative stage, the psychosexologist, thanks to this preliminary work, can enter into the sexuality of the patient, observing its implications and meanings.

And in the end, the psychosexologist can help the patient to reinvest in his manliness, in a "second project of man," as an equal to the rest of the male world.

2.9 Sample Questionnaire for Surgeon-Patient Relationship Evaluation

Proposed by the surgeon to the patient after the last preoperative medical examination and to be checked by the psychosexologist.

When I think about my surgical diagnosis:
(a) I feel lost.
(b) I fear that my family members won't get over the situation.
(c) I am no longer a man.
(d) I have confidence in the surgeon.
I fear most:
(a) Feeling pain
(b) The surgery
(c) Feeling sick
(d) The anesthesia
Surgeon information:
(a) Too scientific
(b) Clear and simple, adapted to my understanding
(c) Clear but I couldn't ask questions
(d) I was too afraid to fully understand
About the hospitalization:
(a) I hope that the nurses will be attentive.
(b) I hope to get out of hospital quickly.
(c) My family (my partner) is very concerned.
(d) I hope that my room is quiet.

On discharge:
(a) I fear that the surgeon will be unreachable.
(b) I hope they give me clear instructions on medication and checkups.
(c) I hope I don't feel too much pain.
(d) I don't want to see my friends until I'm perfectly well.
If followed by a psychosexologist:
(a) I think I can manage by myself.
(b) It would be useful to see the psychosexologist with my partner.
(c) I'm not in a stable sexual relationship.
(d) I'm not sure what a psychosexologist is.

It is not a test but a proposal of questionnaire that may help the meeting between the psychosexologist and the surgeon in the preoperative phase. It is also an instrument of comparison between the ideas of the patient in the preoperative phase and the rehabilitation meeting with the psychosexologist in the postoperative phase. The rest is clinical practice.

References

1. Frank A (1998) Just listening: narrative and deep illness. Fam Syst Health 16(3):197–221
2. Zoppi M (1991) Aspetti psicologici del dolore. In: Mannaioni PF et al (eds) Capire e trattare il dolore. Excepta Medica, Amsterdam
3. Jirojwong S, Manderson L (2002) Physical health and preventive health behaviors among Thai women in Brisbane, Australia. Health Care Women Int 23:197–206

3 The Teenager and His Parents: How Do They Face Andrological Surgery?

If the lack of the maternal figure is one of the main causes of psychic trauma for a child, for the teenager, it is the ambiguity of the messages that come to him from those around him: reassuring on the part of the health care staff, anxiogenic on that of the parents. The teenager, unlike the child, comes into contact with the hospital environment at a time when he is searching for autonomy and sexual identity. The onset of erotic fantasies marks the transition from the intimacy of the child to that of the young adult.

Andrological surgery has therefore a strong influence on the developing male role. He feels depersonalized in an environment with rules and standards at odds with those he is used to, rules that take him away from his peer group, motorcycles, music, video games, tablets, and role-play games on the computer.

The personality of the teenager, which is still developing, offers him a low threshold of frustration and a lack of the stable emotional balance that could make him rationalize the clinical situation.

The "wound" that will be inflicted in the genital area during surgery makes him fear for his life: for the first time, he is afraid of death.

Adolescent males show greater psychological discomfort in the preoperative phase than do females. In fact, manliness is often associated with independence and action, and in these situations, the adolescent may feel socially and sexually inadequate.

In the world of the child, the line between reality and fantasy is not well defined, and, faced with a frightening event, the child can experience fantasies and magical thinking as reality, in order to exorcise the fear.

The level of danger that alerts the teenager is much more conscious; it is real.

Confusion, fear, and sadness are natural responses, which may disappear with the support and the physical and emotional closeness of family members. However, clinical experience shows that preadolescents and adolescents in the pre-surgical phase can have recurrent anxiety attacks, which are anything but transient [1].

E. V. Longhi et al., *Psychosexual Counseling in Andrological Surgery*,
https://doi.org/10.1007/978-3-319-99646-2_3

The most common pathology associated with highly stressful surgical experience is defined post-traumatic stress.

Just as some adults, adolescents have experienced depression, substance abuse, eating disorders, and aggressive and impulsive behavior. For this reason, it is desirable that the parents refrain from expressing concern in front of the child.

The anxiety of a parent, sometimes manifested with overprotective attitudes, or a carefree "we're men, we're not afraid of anything," can increase fears and anxiety about death.

Hard to imagine though it may be, fear is a neutral feeling: a means of encouraging prudence and of selecting the most suitable responses to the clinical situation.

Its physical manifestation however is anything but neutral: pallor, tremors, tachycardia and sometimes even enuresis, apathy, and a sudden lack of interest. There is more. The adolescent is constantly undergoing physiological changes in his search for a new identity: for the first time, he asks clear questions.

"What kind of man do I want to be?"

"How will my body fare in comparison with other males?"

"What price am I willing to pay to become a successful man? (with women)"

Events such as illness, accidents, and surgery make it more difficult to define a body's identity and adolescents may experience:

1. Fear of appearing weak—a teenager may feel uncomfortable with the idea of appearing frightened and fragile or of having childish reactions, such as crying because of painful or unpleasant clinical procedures (application of dressings).
2. Fear of showing his body—having to undress in front of doctors or nurses can be a stressful experience for a teenager, especially when more than one person is present in the room.
3. Fear of being disfigured—the fear of remaining "forever marked, disfigured" by some medical procedure or surgery and of no longer being able to enjoy genital physical integrity.
4. Fear of death—it is common for a teenager, in the construction of their own physical identity and sexual role, to ask questions about life, death, and existence. While hospitalized, this intense fear of death may cause a patient to misinterpret a state of physical fatigue, as a serious sign that the surgery did not go well.

3.1 Risk Factors and Protective Factors

The variables which must be considered in order to understand and prevent distressing situations can be found in the character, temperament, personality, sensitivity, and emotional maturity of the adolescent, as well as in the communication between the parents, their relationship, and within the general family context.

Some factors may increase fear and anguish of death in the adolescent, for example:

1. Previous stressful situations (mourning, change of school or city) and depressive or anxiety disorders prior to surgery
2. Immaturity and poor grasp of reality—where entirely innocuous situations (being in the room with a bigger guy) may be a cause of anxiety, especially for a teenager
3. The presence of deep-rooted convictions—"I'll never get better," "I'm in hospital because I secretly smoked a few joints," etc.
4. Isolation from the family network—from siblings, parents who have separated, the grandfather who got sick, etc.
5. Inability to maintain habits—even eating
6. Being exposed, within the hospital setting, to the sight of blood—injury or other adolescents in a serious condition, who have undergone multiple surgical interventions

Prevention and protection factors:

1. Cognitive factors and personality—the clinical experience shows that sociability and the ability to communicate empathically with adults will be useful in overcoming an ordeal.
2. The real and the emotional age of the adolescent—do not always coincide during the process of the search for identity. A 13-year-old may exhibit the emotional maturity of an 8-year-old, whereas a 12-year-old adolescent may demonstrate the problem-solving skills of a 15-year-old.
3. Familial factors—a reassuring style from one or both parents can ease the anguish of surgery. Single or divorced parents in a state of conflict may on the other hand induce symptoms of anxiety and panic.
4. The friendship and support of school friends—teachers, teammates, and hospital volunteers can raise the stress threshold.
5. Timeliness in reading the emotional discomfort—of both the family and the adolescent is an important psychological factor and is a therapeutic aid both pre- and postoperative.

There is more however. For the benefit of his own mental well-being, the adolescent receives selected information, agreed with the reference figures and according to the principal that not knowing the truth amounts to a more benevolent truth. For some parents, what is unsaid seems to saturate every type of difficult relationship.

The surgeon, at best, talks to the adolescent and to the parents but not always to the siblings.

Unlike children, who in their fear to understand hide their feelings to protect their parents, the adolescent retreats into silence to conceal his anguish at the prospect of death.

Often, complaints about symptoms (not motivated by surgery or by taking medication) are charged with psychological meanings, in the belief that:

"Inside the body there are diseased cells"

"Genitals are deformed"

This action draws the attention of doctors and nurses to the hypothesis of a postoperative complication, for example, and the adolescent transfers to them his fear of understanding, and of knowing, so that his life becomes extraneous to him and that in time someone will take responsibility for it.

3.2 Siblings of the Patient

During the diagnostic and presurgical phases, the patient's siblings are almost ignored as attention is focused instead on anxiety and fear of the surgical procedure (fini, [2]).

At first, the siblings develop defense mechanisms to withstand the emergence of such family anguish and come to the hospital mostly after surgery, because clinically most has been done.

At this stage the family begins to think about future projects and take care of necessities and the needs of the other children. The healthy siblings begin to show feelings of fear, anger, and rebellion.

They appear irritable at school and aggressive toward parents, exhibiting symptoms of dermatosis, gastric reflux, headaches, and insomnia. The siblings seem unconscious to choose the same communication as the hospitalized adolescent, that is, through the body, perhaps believing that only by being sick can they attract healthy attention, without feeling any sense of guilt.

And then, who understands that in such instances to be "healthy" is a responsibility and perhaps even a fault?

"at home you don't count for anything, rather, because you are healthy you mustn't cause any problems. You absolutely must do well at school and in sport, go out little with friends, because you will hear that you are selfish..." (the rant of a twin brother aged 15 years)

"...then if you are female, everything is expected. As mum is always at the hospital with my brother, everyone assumes that at 17 I can replace my mother. Try telling your boyfriend to understand the situation…and my dad asks 'have you heard from your mother?' and me?..." (the outburst of an elder sister)

Such manifestations seem to be a way to communicate through the body "we are here, we won't abandon you, we won't betray you." On the other hand, they seek, in rancor and anger, a bond with the hospitalized brother and the parents.

In the interview with the siblings, the psychosexologist often draws a circle and begins:

> *Let us assume that this circle is the relational space of your family. Mark the places occupied by your hospitalized brother, your parents and you within the circle. (a systemic instrument known as "relationship space")*

Usually, the hospitalized brother is placed in the center of the circle, close to the parents. The siblings place themselves on the outer edge of the circle, or worse they do not draw at all.

Being healthy is in these situations an uncomfortable truth, almost an injustice:

"You feel like a survivor. Everyone expects twice as much of everything from you, for you to look out for two (for you and your brother), not to cause bother and problems, to be an adult for two or three or four (for you, your brother and your parents)."

3.3 What to Report to the Medical Team?

The close collaboration between clinicians, surgeons, and the psychosexologist determines not only the healing process but also the process of care for the patient and his family.

The need for an integrated diagnostic and therapeutic approach, which takes account of patients' suffering and history, in terms of complexity should be the premise of the surgical approach and of the psychosexologist.

The surgeon and the psychosexologist presenting themselves together promote a global evaluation of the patient and accelerate the therapeutic contract between these three individuals.

Working as a team with the nursing staff offers a chance to see the disease in terms of clinical, emotional, and relational complexity, both in the team (the way operator feels in front of the teenager and his family) and in relationship with the patient and family.

The more authentic the integration (how much every clinician is able to observe the patient as a whole person, not just through the severity of the disease), the sooner the healing team will establish a therapeutic contract of respect, trust, and collaboration with the adolescent and in the family context.

This creates a positive circular relationship of encouragement and engagement and the easy solution of emotional, relational, and clinical difficulties.

The psychosexologist works simultaneously both within the clinical team and in following the patient and his family relationships.

An ad hoc facilitator who from time to time involves the patient, the parents and the siblings and puts them in touch with the care team while respecting each individual professional competence.

On this basis of trust, the psychosexologist may enter into the intimacy of the adolescent and accommodate him with regard to his doubts, anguish, and fragility, helping him, in confidence, to regain a sexual role more suited to a young man's life.

3.4 The Parental Anxiety

Parental anxieties are varied and individual. Among the most common are observing your son in a state of helplessness, dealing with his first surgical experience, having an only child, working in health care, the severity of the surgery, and separation from the teenager before anesthesia.

Furthermore: the lack of a well-defined role during surgery.

In this regard, one study has shown that if the parent is free to choose a technique to reduce tension in the son, the level of anxiety of family members is reduced, because the parents thereby acquire a mechanism to control the anguish of separation [3].

Everyday clinical experience suggests that showing a film or drawing the parent a diagram of the type of surgical procedure the child will undergo can increase the understanding of family members and share the clinical path with the child.

In addition, many family members show prejudice toward anesthesia, foreseeing difficulty when the child comes round, for example, nausea and vomiting. There is also the painful prospect that the child could die during surgery.

The need to share in the surgeon's responsibility for the surgical path leads many parents to accuse the doctor of lacking openness, of holding back information, and of not understanding their need for attention and to know, above all, about anesthesia.

Two types of parents have been identified:

1. The family with an internal locus of control asks details even weeks and months before the child's operation to establish their own strategies for coping.
2. The family with an external locus of control requires only a limited amount of information, to safeguard against anxiety.

Even day surgery does not improve parents' states of anxiety, which often unwittingly and not a little counteract adolescents' compliance, nullifying their physical and emotional improvements during home convalescence.

One positive factor is the lower level of cortisol present in the parent accompanying the patient than that found in other family members. It is usually the mother who spends most time visiting in hospital, often accompanying the child as far as the operating theatre.

According to a study, when the father is present, the stress level of the adolescent is higher, probably because of the importance of the caring role attributed to the mother in Mediterranean culture.

Finally, it seems that parents generally have low expectations regarding the behavior of the pre- and postoperative teenager, often describing him as shy or particularly nervous in stressful situations or in contact with strangers:

"I know him: he would cry in stressful situations, he becomes more and more nervous ... anxious. "even in a basketball tournament ..." (the mother of a 14-year-old boy)

Or that previous bad experiences with his healthcare professional can adversely affect the emotions of her son:

"...he passed out during a blood test and has been afraid of needles ever since. The nurses always have to calm him down. For him though, it's a trauma every time ... how will he get over the surgery?..." (father of a 12-year-old boy)

3.5 Returning Home

As much as it is desired, even returning home can be difficult for a teenager: anger, sadness, aggression, and impatience may be more evident than during hospitalization.

At home, the adolescent rediscovers his old habits and his security, so he can be freer to express repressed resentments and anxieties, particularly toward parents, because they are ready to understand him and not deprive him of emotional support.

The following reactions might present:

- A low attention span
- Changes in sleep-wake rhythms or changes in eating habits
- Frequent temper tantrums, anger and fear
- Hyperactivity or apathy, lack of interest, chronic fatigue
- Presence of worries and fears that prevent the adolescent resuming school activity and/or sport
- Appearance of new and persistent fears
- Total rejection of study and school
- Complete loss of interest in friends and social activities
- Conflict with siblings, friends, parents

3.6 Conclusions

Andrological surgery is performed on still developing, sensitive patients on the road to sexual maturity. Wounding to the genital area reveals the anguish of death and causes the boy to think about life and existence in a deep and conscious manner.

Brothers, sisters, and family members, when under stress, build sometimes contradictory and complex relationships.

The surgeon and the psychosexologist can, side by side, decode these processes and construct individualized diagnostic and surgical procedures every time.

References

1. Caprilli S, Messeri A (2004) Il dolore nel bambino: aspetti clinici, psicologici e principali elementi di trattamento. In: Gioffrè D (ed) Il dolore non necessario. Prospettive medico-sanitarie e culturali. Bollati Boringhieri, Torino
2. Paolucci G (2002) Anxiety, stress and preoperative surgical nursing. Prof Inferm 3:180–191
3. Kain ZN et al (2003) Parental intervention choices for children undergoing repeated surgeries. Anesth Analg 96:970–975

4 LGBT Families

Homosexuality is not incompatible with parenting. According to the Italian National Health Institute, there are more than 100,000 homosexual parents, 300,000 in France, 400,000 in Spain, and between 7 and 16 million in the United States, not to mention the rest of the world.

Even today, there are two types of worries and often a cultural inadequacy, even on the part of clinicians:

1. The first concerns the compatibility between homosexuality and parental function.
2. The second concerns the possibility for a teenager to grow up "healthy" where the parents are a same-sex couple and above all the ability to differentiate between roles and sexual identity. Will he/she have more difficulty?

Excluding ethical-religious, political-cultural, legal, and political-religious approaches, the surgeon and psychosexologist can only turn to the evidence of scientific studies that to date number more than one hundred. Referenze molto datate

Greenfel [1] confirmed that the reasons for parenting are the same for both same-sex and heterosexual couples. However, achieving the goal of parenting can be a much greater medical and psychological effort for same-sex couples, due to both social prejudice and the fact that, unlike heterosexual couples, homogenous couples do not enjoy the same support from their families of origin, friends, and the social network in general.

Thirty-five international studies [2] have confirmed there is a high psychosocial risk of depression among young lesbian, gay, and bisexual people.

Among the main factors are stress from hiding and managing a socially stigmatized identity, rejection by the parents, abuse and other traumatic events, negative interpersonal interactions, and school bullying. As a result, young same-sex

E. V. Longhi et al., *Psychosexual Counseling in Andrological Surgery*,
https://doi.org/10.1007/978-3-319-99646-2_4

parents may face a number of threats to their mental health. Surgeon and psychosexologist cannot deny this evidence and omit to observe the effects on the adolescent patient.

More specifically, Borghi (2009) proposed a classification of homogeneous (same sex) typologies according to the structure criterion:

1. Lesbian or gay families: these are families in which two women decide to have a child using the seed of a donor or two men decide to have a child using "surrogacy".
2. Homoricompound families: these are households made up of, for example, two women or two men, one of whom has had a child from an earlier heterosexual relationship or a single lesbian mother who finds a partner.
3. Families with an enlarged constitution: these are tetrageneral families in which two couples, one gay and one lesbian, decide to cooperate to have a child. The child will be biologically linked to one member of each of the two couples, but all four will share the role of parent. Finally, there are triparental families in which a couple collaborates with a single person who maintains his or her parental function.
4. Single-parent family: where the parent, usually a woman, remains single.

Investigating each of these forms of LGBT parenting entails tracing the same results as follows:

> ...there is no evidence that lesbian women or gay men are not suited to becoming parents or that psychosocial development among the children of lesbian women or gay men, when compared with that of the children of heterosexual parents, is compromised..... To date, evidence suggests that the domestic environment created by homosexual parents is as likely to support and realize the psychosocial development of their children as that of heterosexual parents....

It would seem that the assumption that a parent of the same sex, as the reference model, is needed to bring out the role and sexual identity of the child and that a parent of the opposite sex is needed to verify it has been dropped.

Some questions however remain open:

1. The internal relationship of the lesbian or gay couple, their capacity to mediate, conflict resolution.
2. The management of relationships with the extended family, before and after the arrival of children.
3. The choice of donor.
4. The choice of the role of the donor, who will have constructed a relationship with the parents during the 9 months of gestation.
5. What answers to give the child about difficulties in comparison with the social context and the mistakes to avoid?
6. The emotivity and psyche of the non-biological parent in the face of frustration at the lack of a socially accepted role.

7. How are the roles of non-biological parents divided within same sex partnerships?
8. What kind of educational relationship will the former heterosexual partner set up in the new homosexual family?

Questions on which there is still debate even today and on which the surgeon and the psychosexologist can only hope to avoid criticism and judgment.

The analysis of family themes must be a premise for welcoming and accompanying the patient and his or her family, whatever its composition, not denying its characteristics, dynamics, and peculiarities.

4.1 Children of Same-Sex Couples

If we refer to the sexual development of children of LGBT families, studies confirm that they develop in a similar way to children of heterosexual families, especially with regard to sexual orientation, sexual role, and the relationship with male and female cultural models.

With respect to childhood and adolescence, it would seem that the children of LGBT parents have a better outlook regarding their professional future and the males show a lower level of aggressiveness.

These young people also show a greater openness to the possibility of discovering themselves non-heterosexual; psychoaffective research does not reveal any relevance to depressive anxious symptoms or symptoms of social phobia.

Hall's studies [2] show how these children, at around the age of 6, can show more insecurity and less self-esteem, perhaps linked to having fewer models of comparison with other peers (compared to children with heterosexual parents), which can create a sense of being different and loneliness.

The same study shows that by around the age of 12 this insecurity has almost disappeared, while by the age of 18/19 the same children find themselves with greater self-esteem and less hostility than their peers.

This might lead one to think of a supposed greater social competence, caused by having learned to be part of a minority and having to explain to the majority of peers who you are and how you behave in relationships.

There is more. LGBT families are well aware of the social discrimination that their children will have to face and are able to put in place a series of procedures to alert teachers and social workers from kindergarten onward [3].

We are therefore dealing with families who are open with and visible to teachers and educators. They are keen to offer them information and relationship details in order to improve integration with classmates (children with heterosexual parents) and the adults in the scholastic world, precisely so that their peculiarity is not ignored.

This avoids a standardized pedagogy limiting itself to addressing a heterosexual majority, at odds with the minority group of children with LGBT families.

4.2 About the Donor

As for the relationship with the figure of the donor (in same-sex female families who use heterologous medically assisted procreation), data from the National Longitudinal Lesbian Family Study suggest that curiosity about the donor is greater when the child is given the opportunity to contact him and meet him on reaching the age of 18.

Other studies suggest that curiosity is linked to the possibility of giving a face to the donor, along with the telling of family stories, verifying the physical similarities, to enable the construction of a father-child relationship, above all for future development.

The surgeon and the psychosexologist, by discussing these family systems, can share a path of self-learning and reinvest these skills in a confrontation between cultural prejudices and individual sensitivities.

The sexuality of the children of same-sex parent families shows a complexity of references and educational models that are invaluable for the care of the young patient and in preventing surgical and behavioral complications during the stay.

4.3 Conclusions

The same-sex parent family must be scrutinized in all roles and relationships: starting from the child's inner world and the development of his or her identity and needs and moving on to the parents and their personal history.

In the andrological surgical experience, all these worlds become disturbed with regard to security and sexual identity. Following the young patient of homosexual parents triggers the curiosity of the psychosexologist as to the process of identity and sexual role without comparison with other young people of heterosexual parents.

In the same way, the medical team must be educated, albeit through the sensitivity of the psychosexologist, to examine their own prejudices and difficulties of comparison.

References

1. Greenfel DA (2016) Playing a homosexual: medical treatment and psychosocial considerations. Curr Opin Obstet Gynecol 28(3):202–209
2. Hall WJ (2018) Psychosocial risk and protective factors for depression among young lesbians, gays, bisexuals, queers: a systematic review. J Homosex 65(3):263–316
3. Goldberg AE et al (2018) Meet other moms: adoptive mothers lesbian relationships with other parents at school and not only. J Lesbian Stud 22(1):67–84

Body Image: What Does It Tell the Andrologist Surgeon?

5

Whenever the body and skin are affected by andrological (typically pelvic) surgery, the body image of the individual is damaged, and we cannot avoid seeing particular characteristics.

Why? The development of body image is a very delicate process that begins in the womb. In this period, the child has a symbiotic bond with the mother, through which it feels her emotions and feelings, perceiving them as if they were his/her own.

Thus, also his bodily boundaries are those of the mother. At birth, the newborn baby has no feeling of self, no perception of his body and its constituent parts. The newborn experiences legs, arms, head and neck as foreign parts, not integrated with each other.

During the first 3 years, the child refines the ability to distinguish itself from others and perceives his or her body as a whole while distinguishing the individual parts and their functions.

From 4 to 6 years of age, the child experiences a growing mobility that allows him/her to consciously acquire the sensations of the body and of the relationship between the body and the outside world.

Around the age of 6, the child is able to articulate his or her actions in an increasingly complex way, acquiring a distinct perception of right and left, front and back, and high and low.

From 7 to 12 years old, the ability to abstract appears, allowing the formation of the mental image of one's own body. In the development of body image, the primary relationship of attachment plays a fundamental role.

The mother in fact represents the intermediary between the child and the outside world. The look from the figure of attachment represents for the little one his/her first emotional recognition as a "lovable individual."

Pietropolli Charmet [1] hypothesizes that the individual with body image disorders may have had experiences of disconfirmation in the mother's gaze that have damaged his/her ability to love and to be loved.

E. V. Longhi et al., *Psychosexual Counseling in Andrological Surgery*,
https://doi.org/10.1007/978-3-319-99646-2_5

In practice, the mother, not finding her aesthetic ideal in her son's beauty, questions the emotional relationship. The quality and quantity of emotional-relational exchanges between mother and child would have a determining influence on the perception and construction of the patient's body image.

In this way physical contact with the child, language, and tone of voice provide the child with important information about what it is like, what its body is like, and what its relationship is with the outside world.

This is where the definition of the child's body image begins, from the positive features (accepted by the mother) to the negative, which are a long way from the mother's aesthetic-emotional expectations.

How can this premise not be taken into account in an andrological and psychosexual anamnesis?

5.1 Everything There Is to Know

According to Cash's model of social cognitive learning [2], the development of body image is influenced by four factors:

1. Physical
2. Sociocultural
3. Psychological
4. Interpersonal

The observation of one's own body and how it compares with social models of physical adequacy or inadequacy (build, height, etc.) becomes the reference values of every individual when it comes to feeling confirmed or disconfirmed with regard to external physical appearance.

Moreover, according to Festinger [3], the tendency toward comparison with other people develops skills, abilities, and qualities of prestige over others (muscular body, blue eyes, etc.) or, on the other hand, feelings of uneasiness and being less appealing than one's peers (being excessively underweight and overweight or being of only average height).

5.1.1 Physical Factors

Two of the most important variables are the weight and muscle tone of the body, because they influence attractiveness, allure, and social desirability, not forgetting the influence of the concomitant cultural, social, and family prejudices.

Unlike women, for whom standards of slimness play a fundamental role in the perception of body image, men are more interested in the function of their bodies: for example, how well the body performs physically, the quality of erection during sexual intercourse.

5.1.2 Sociocultural Factors

"Who am I as a body?"

"How do I feel in relation to others?"

These are the terms of comparison of one's own body image with the models of attractiveness learned from the media and from the process of individual internalization of such models.

In answer to the question "How do you see yourself?", one 13-year-old replied.

A frog. I am short and stick thin and the only thing I can do to be better than anyone else is athletics (running).

"I like to eat and even the doctor (andrologist) said that I have to slim down. I'm a 'balloon'," replied a young man of 15.

"Girls don't like me and now I'm sick too and they're going to operate on my penis…. "

Parents, siblings, sisters, and relatives in general (and all the reference persons of each individual) then play a fundamental role in the formation of body image.

Comments, jokes, and criticisms about body image affect the individual for a long time:

> … as a child I was shy, pale and with few muscles, unlike my brother. 'He's an athlete.' my father told me, and from that day on I started boxing. Today, at 45 years of age, I am a competition judge, as a hobby, in junior boxing matches….

as can the message of how much the body can be an important reference to living the right way, thinking appropriately, and having an amiable manner.

"You never see your father going out of the house scruffy, without shaving and with messy hair? Follow his example… that's what my mother said then," reports a 32-year-old man.

"And today. Have a look in the mirror, do you look alright?… and to think that I made you so beautiful…."

The peer group plays a similar role to the family environment. The group's opinions (in relation to weight, body shape, height, etc.) are learned as models to be aimed at and adhered to.

Recent studies [4] have shown that having one's leg pulled about physical appearance has a greater impact on children and adolescents than on adults.

There is more however.

5.1.3 Psychological Factors

All these models and all this conditioning are mediated by the psychological characteristics of the individual, the level of self-esteem, and the idea of how body image can further add value to or debase the individual.

The relationship between self-esteem and body image is very complex. In males, for example, one of the main sources of pride is the progressive increase in muscle mass alongside the shape and size of the penis.

Many studies confirm the correlation between low self-esteem and body dissatisfaction, especially in adolescents [5].

In the same way, the personality traits most dependent on body image pertain to a narcissistic and hyper-perfectionist personality. These characteristics predispose the person to make assessments and opinions on their physical appearance, which are, for the most part, negative.

This type of personality can become pathological, especially in the context of andrological surgery because the individual has a strong investment in himself and in the conventions of bodily perfection.

The need for admiration and hypersensitivity to criticism in such people are defensive mechanisms, used to conceal a fragile self-esteem. Under-assessing or underestimating them could lead the patient to dysfunctional behavior at the expense of successful andrological surgery.

Also, the sense of grandeur of which such personalities are possessed produces an idea of their own perfect body image, far removed from reality.

Consequently, even a perfectly successful surgery from both the clinical and aesthetic points of view can become an element of failure in the patient if he feels adversely affected by sexual performance expectations and his own virility.

This failure may have a strong impact on body image and become a premise for further sexual and eating disorders and alcohol addiction.

5.1.4 Interpersonal Factors

Many studies then focused on sexual and emotional relations. Being in a satisfactory loving relationship and feeling attractive to one's partner become an element of confirmation and approval of one's own body image.

On the other hand, incidences of rejection can affect not only body image but also the sense of pleasure and cause subsequent failures in sexual experiences during the various ages of development. The individual will be led to associate sexual experiences with shame and embarrassment, rejecting them a priori or renouncing their own bodily pleasure (e.g., ejaculation disorders).

Many people in adulthood remember andrological surgery in adolescence as a:

> Dramatic event and a source of pain and the feeling of being a victim of violence. I could have kept my varicocele, I told myself, when I observed my swollen penis. I'm finished, I thought…. today with my partner I can't stand oral sex or being touched on the penis… (Adrian, 38 years old).

5.2 Body Image and Gender Identity

From the moment the body undergoes transformations in terms of weight, height, body mass, and the development of secondary sexual characteristics, the cultural expectations associated with physical appearance gradually change.

The male body, particularly in its aesthetic aspect, becomes the instrument through which to express and project ideals of virility, dominance, power, strength, and control. In this context, teenagers and adults often amplify these characteristics through bodybuilding, diet, and the intake of substances that support muscle development (proteins, vitamins, anabolic steroids) with sometimes dangerous and morbid effects on health.

Every individual invests in his/her gender identity behaviors, attitudes, and ways of thinking which enable the accentuation of the ego, in a process of growth dating back to the first 12–18 months of life, which leads the individual to perceive himself/herself, to characterize his/her gender, and to improve sexual performance and powers of seduction.

5.3 Conclusion

The sexological anamnesis cannot therefore disregard examination of the body image and the sexual identity connected to it. Gender identity is, in fact, linked to the perception we have of our bodies.

Uncertainties regarding sexual identity or difficulty in accepting one's sexual identity (e.g., homosexuality, latent, or otherwise) may be the reasons for a change in body image perception.

Body shapes which are considered unattractive will clash with the objectives of health, aesthetics, and pleasure that every surgeon strives to achieve in order to optimize the quality of life of the patient, especially in adolescence.

The psychosexologist then provides those observations that allow the surgeon and the medical team to parameterize their clinical intent with the style of personality of the patient and, if this is pathological or heavily altered, to advise against, if possible, an intervention that would be a further cause of frustration, inadequacy, and social marginalization.

References

1. Charmet P (2013) La paura di essere brutti. Cortina, Milano
2. Cash TF (2011) Cognitive behavioral perspectives on body image. In: Cash et al (eds) Body image: a handbook of science. Practice and prevention, 2nd edn. Guilford Press, New York
3. Festinger L (1954) A theory of social comparison processes. Hum Relat 7:117–140
4. Carlson JD (2012) Body image: peer Influences. In: Encyclopedia of body image and human appearance. Elsevier, London
5. O'Dea JA (2012) Body image and self esteem. In: Encyclopedia of body image and human appearance. Elsevier, London

6 Identity Card: Body Image Diagnosis

The body, a source of adequacy and self-esteem or inadequacy and dissatisfaction, is the focus of the individual's thoughts, as well as of evaluation by psychiatrists, andrologists, and psychosexologists.

A study by Jafferany [1] assessed body parts that worry teenagers with male body dysmorphic disorder (BDD): 35% were concerned about facial features, 17.6% about the skin (color, any marks, moles, scars), 30% about lips (shape, size, dimensions), 18% about teeth (size, color), 6% about ears and eyes (size, color, shape), and 58% about the penis (shape, size, color).

Body dysmorphism is in fact a disorder of the body image that obsessively highlights the defects of its aesthetic aspect, to the point of compromising the social, scholastic, or work sphere of the patient.

In this sense, a request for penis lengthening, for example, could prove to be an illusory desire for perfection that the andrologist surgeon is not always able to discern a priori.

Even if she/he guesses that certain personality characteristics of the patient appear discordant and contradictory. Hence the help of psychosexological counselling.

What do we find in the course of the sexological anamnesis?

First of all, thoughts about the body (e.g., penis size) are very intrusive for the individual and occupy his mind to the point of obsession for up to 3–8 h a day. The patient assumes that he will be rejected by everyone and everything, because his appearance is considered horrendous, abnormal, and repugnant.

> I have a feeling of disgust when I think about my body, I have terrifying defects and I repulse myself (Gerard, 17 years old).

E. V. Longhi et al., *Psychosexual Counseling in Andrological Surgery*,
https://doi.org/10.1007/978-3-319-99646-2_6

In addition to such thoughts, dysmorphia is characterized by repetitive behaviors that the patient puts in place for most of the day, such as the following:

1. Comparing their own body image with that of other people, including actors and film stars or models in fashion magazines
2. Checking their reflection in front of any mirror, display case, or reflecting surface
3. Asking for external reassurance on their physical appearance in an annoying and repetitive way
4. Continuous requests to doctors for corrective and cosmetic surgery, especially in the pelvic and genital areas

Requests for penis enlargement and remodeling are therefore no exception.

Unlike in Eastern culture, where the identity of the person and his body are one, in the Western world, the body is often alienated from identity, causing a pathological split between the soma, the psyche, and the individual.

Let's take a look.

6.1 Body Dysmorphic Disorders

6.1.1 Bigorexia

Bigorexia or muscle dysmorphophobia has as its main characteristic in the excessive concern for the muscular mass and causes perceptive, affective, and behavioral disorders that interfere with everyday life. In the world of bodybuilding is found mostly in subjects between the ages of 15 and 23.

Pope [2] has proposed some evaluation criteria:

1. Concern at not being muscular enough
2. The continuous monitoring of physical appearance in front of any mirror
3. Obsessive attention to diet
4. The use of anabolic steroids

Males with this disease don't worry about being overweight but about having a very low-fat mass perception:

"If I don't go to the gym every day," reports Antony, 16 years old, "I feel swollen and not very toned. I eat less and measure muscle mass. I have to reach 100 kilos to have the muscles I want."

At the root of these pathological ideals lie traits of perfectionism, fear of maturity, inadequacy, and a drive toward a prolonged and perennial adolescence.

How can this not be taken into account in the run up to andrological surgery?

6.1.2 Tanorexia

Tanorexia is a body obsession that concerns the degree of tanning of the skin: the patient obsessively exposes himself/herself to the sun's rays or attends specialized solariums daily.

In this disease, the individual's feeling of insecurity would be overcome by an attractive, exotic body image, with which he/she is never satisfied.

6.1.3 Masculine Anorexia Nervosa

Masculine anorexia nervosa is certainly the most known pathology while being the most insidious, tenacious, and deadly.

The diagnostic features described in DSM-5 report are the following:

1. Excessively low body weight, taking into account the parameters of height, sex, developmental path, and physical and mental health.

> My ideal weight is 38 kg. I am 1.70 tall and I hate any kind of protruding fat.... I weigh myself every day and my dance teacher is the only one who supports me. Everyone is against me. They don't have my self-control regarding food and every time I see them giving in, I triumph as if on stage... (Federich, 15 years old).

2. Intense fear of gaining weight or becoming fat, with strict rules on fasting.
3. The ideal body weight and shape are the basis of the individual's level of self-esteem, to the point of ignoring the risks of being underweight.

Abstinence from food also extends to sexual desire, to the drives of pleasure. All sensations are anesthetized in a sort of limbo, where what counts is rigor, absolute control and perfectionism in the achievement of professional and scholastic goals. Being *top of the class* is the norm even among friends and in all social contexts.

The persistence of the pathology is often aggravated by the reactions of family members [3] who, in an effort to counter the self-destructive behavior of their relative, involuntarily engage in a real power struggle.

> The more obsessive they are about watching my plate, the more I lose appetite and the fight then spreads to everything. Every doctor they meet seeks allies. Every opportunity is a taken to repeat that I am always tense and that I no longer have the stamina I had when I was in bloom... (Arthur, 17 years old).

Bearing this in mind, andrological surgery requires an a priori contract with the patient. It is agreed with him that during the hospital stay, nobody will make him put on weight. In return, he will have to agree with the doctors on a more suitable diet for surgery, hospitalization, and the resumption of school, sports, and musical activities.

The psychosexologist will act as a guarantor and facilitator in communications with doctors and nurses. In a second phase, focusing on the patient's sense of perfectionism, he will be invited to post-op interviews to reinvest with him emotions, fears, feelings of hatred, stress, and depression, in a (therapeutic) context that guarantees professional secrecy. Without mentioning food, rather relationships, confrontation with others: the real difficulties of the patient [4].

6.1.4 Bulimia Nervosa

Bulimia nervosa, on the other hand, is a pathology that leads patients to an uncontrollable need for food and anxious ingestion of any comestibles, without experiencing the flavor and the resulting pleasure.

> I wake up at night with strong anxiety and a hole in my stomach. I have to eat at all costs and alone, without the others (family members) seeing me. I eat everything I find in the refrigerator… once I ate frozen ravioli because I couldn't stop myself anymore… (Alfred, 14 years old).

The diagnostic criteria for bulimia nervosa reported in DSM-5 regard:

1. Compulsively eating a quantity of food (up to 5000 calories) that exceeds every standard
2. Inability to stop eating or to control the quality of food ingested
3. Compensatory rituals to prevent weight gain, such as self-induced vomiting, laxative abuse, diuretics, and excessive exercise

> …for three years I've been vomiting, even in fast food restaurants. But it is increasingly difficult to do so. My jaws are sore…now a friend of mine has told me to drink balsamic vinegar and in a short time vomiting is induced… (Louis, 16 years old).

Levels of self-esteem in these patients are influenced by the weight and shape of their dry and mostly dehydrated body. This disease does not necessarily appear after episodes of anorexia and in the male population is also a source of an ideal stereotyped strength, of omnipotent virility.

These patients do not engage in exhausting physical activities, nor do they resort to corrective measures (laxatives, vomiting) against weight gain.

They overestimate their physical and emotional strength: how should we proceed?

Only by relying on the sense of solitude of such conduct can a therapeutic contract of trust be obtained, provided the patient's trust is not betrayed and is not abandoned after hospital discharge:

> *(the psychosexologist) I don't know how you keep everything to yourself. Not asking for help, not sharing with someone…I don't know, you seem very alone and I don't know how many people realize your silent suffering….*

(Henry 17 years old)...I'm sorry (he cries), it took me by surprise...I'm afraid of disappointing, of worrying my family...there's no place for me at home. Adele (his 14-year-old sister who has Down's syndrome) needs attention and I try to make her laugh, but I often feel so much anxiety and sadness. Is it normal?

6.1.5 Binge Eating Disorder

Binge eating disorder, on the other hand, is characterized by recurrent episodes of binge eating of at least 2 h once a week.

This is followed by feelings of frustration, unease, inadequacy and guilt, not least because these behaviors are more frequent in people who are overweight and on diets. Cash et al. [5] showed that obese people, old and young, even if losing weight, do not achieve a stable and positive body image but maintain problems of control, insecurity, and low self-esteem.

All of which makes it easy to deduce that these disorders connected to body image are more cognitive, affective, and psychic than physical.

6.2 What Lies Behind Body Dysmorphism?

Clinical experience shows that in every type of bodily dysmorphism, there lie a major depressive disturbance, social phobia, anxiety, perfectionism, low self-esteem, and extroversion.

Investigating the body image of preoperative patients means assessing emotional aspects, the patient's family history, pain threshold, individual compliance, mood swings, emotional fragility, and life motivation.

Not all adolescent and adult patients see themselves projected, after surgery, into a world of plans and opportunities. Often the fear of failure and of assuming roles of maturity induces adolescents with body dysmorphism to "make of disease," the most reassuring life project.

Post-surgical, psychosomatic and emotional symptoms appear to be disguised requests for help seeking guidance in life.

"I'm fine with doctors. You listen to me, you don't treat me like a child. You understand that I'm gambling more than my virility," exclaims Marck, 15 years old, "out there, (the world) everyone pretends. But what do they know about me? Can't I be afraid without being criticized?"

Less frequently, these patients show schizoaffective disorders with disorganized behaviors and thoughts. In such cases, psychiatrists and psychosexologists use self-report tests and questionnaires. Among the most used are the following:

1. **BCS (Body Cathexis Scale)**—A 46-item test that assesses dissatisfaction with various parts of the body AND functionality (energy level, taste in clothes, etc).
2. **BIAQ (Body Image Avoidance Questionnaire)**—Assesses the frequency of food control, social activity, weight control and body care, and choice of clothes.

3. **BCQ (Body Checking Questionnaire)**—Detects the frequency of control behavior regarding the body and the patient's aversion to his soma.
4. **Physical Appearance State and Trait Anxiety Scale**—Measures the state of anxiety the patient feels toward parts of his body.
5. **ASI-R (Appearance Schemas Inventory Revised)**—Assesses the power that the patient attributes to his body and his investment in body care image.
6. **BDDQ (Body Dysmorphic Disorder Questionnaire)**—The Body Dysmorphic Disorder Examination (BDDE) is a semi-structured clinical interview designed to diagnose dysmorphic disorder of the body and to measure the symptoms of a severely negative body image. It includes concerns about and negative assessments of appearance, self-awareness and embarrassment, the overemphasis placed on appearance in self-assessment, avoidance of activity, disguise of the body, and body control. BDDE, related to body image measurements, negative self-esteem, and psychological symptoms, was sensitive to change following treatment of dysmorphic body disorder. It has provided unique information in predicting clinical status when controlling psychological adjustment and other measures of body image.

These tools can be followed by a semi-structured interview with BISI—body image structured interview—which evaluates the interpretation of male and female roles, social expectations, the relationship with one's own body, the influence of the media, and the power that the individual attributes to his own body.

Relating with dysmorphic patients means facing a series of emotional defenses that individuals have created over time to protect themselves from the suffering caused by those parts of the body which make them feel inadequate, insecure, fragile, anxious, depressed, and self-destructive.

6.3 Body Map

In addition to questionnaires and structured interviews, the psychosexologist asks the patient to complete his body map during the counselling.

What does it consist of? The patient is given two printed drawings (not all people have artistic skills) of the male body structure, one for the front and one for the back.

He is given three colors to draw areas of pleasure (in red), pain (in blue), and nuisance (in green) on the body in the map.

He is asked.

"What feeling do you want to start with?"

Case History

In Fig. 6.1 is shown the body map designed by 22-year-old Marck, a student at the Faculty of Medicine, who asked the andrologist surgeon for penis lengthening. The patient has a dysmorphic disorder.

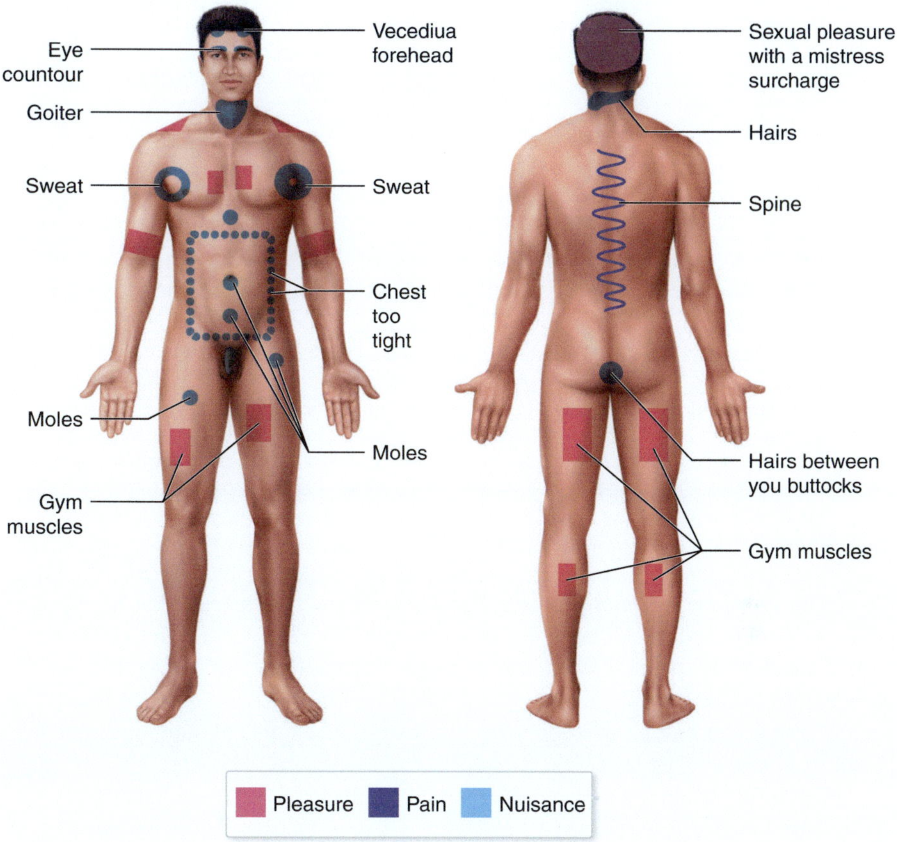

Fig. 6.1

"When I look at myself I'm disgusted"

"How did you get to this feeling?" (psychosexologist)

"You don't know, but as a child I was underweight, the pediatrician said I was only thin, but I saw the other children. The general practitioner told my parents that everything would change with adolescence, but I knew that I had no muscles. Only my psychiatrist, at 17, told me that I was right."

"How did you turn to a psychiatrist?"

"I messed up. I tried to commit suicide because a girl had left me, but now I wouldn't. I am used to occasionally do strange things, especially when I get nervous...."

Marck comments on the sensations of pleasure:

> I feel pleasure when I touch my muscles. I'm a body builder and today I'm 97 kg lean. When I reach 100 kg. I'll be the ideal weight, like the actor Schwarzenegger, my idol.

He adds that he has been taking steroids, anabolic agents, and protein supplements, and in the morning he drinks a smoothie with at least six egg whites, fruit, almonds, carnitine, arginine, and omega-3. The diet is hyper-protein and he trains daily. He caresses his biceps while talking and reports that he experiences a feeling of well-being.

The other sensations of pleasure are linked to meetings with escorts:

> after the end of the affair with that girl, I only looked for escorts. They don't leave me, they don't abandon me and I don't see them only for sex, we talk. They tell me, that I kiss well. To Matilde, the escort I fell in love with today, I asked straight out, 'do you think I have a body that sucks?' She said no. I don't see her as much as I would like. We often get in touch and every time she says 'study!' And I wouldn't want her to treat me like a puppy, I'm fine with her….

The nuisance areas are more demanding. Marck complains that he has a narrow chest and is still not muscular enough. He cannot stand the moles on his chest; they disgust him. He mapped the moles, and everything was negative.

"I even had one on my upper lip, but using the excuse of shaving, I cut it off. Can you see the scar?"

He cannot stand the hairs on the back of his neck and between his buttocks: he depilates every week, especially when he sees Matilde. He is annoyed by sweat, his goiter or Adam's apple, his receding hairline, and the outline of his eyes.

"There is a lot to do," he exclaims and then claims that the only pain he feels is in his spine, because he lifts 60 kg doing weights.

> *"How do you see yourself in the drawing?"* (psychosexologist)

"with Matilde well, I just have to be with her and I feel stronger, more virile. In the drawing I am nervous, depressed, anxious."

Marck then talks about the penis:

> Have you ever seen an erect penis in a porn film? they're at least 30 cm. I'm not talking about that size, but my request is normal….

> *"What does Matilde say about your genitals?"* (psychosexologist)

"She says I'm normal"

"And isn't that enough for you? Why should Matilde lie to you?" (psychosexologist)

"No, Matilde is sincere, but if I look at myself… However a friend of mine has given me a good idea. When I get to 100 kg of muscle mass, he asked me to strip in gay clubs for money. I don't know them, so …."

What comes to light? Since childhood, Marck has spoken with psychiatrists and therapists. He needs to speak, to reassure himself, and the female world frightens him.

Penis lengthening is just a way to seem important among the specialists and therapists. He is aware of his dysmorphism, he was told about it by the psychiatrist at 17 years of age, and they often spoke about the aesthetic ideal at Schwarzenegger. He may be a doctor, but he fears blood and diseases. In the anatomy I exam, he says, they asked him to extract the eyeballs from a corpse, and he fainted.

- Marck has an older brother with whom he does not speak. He becomes red in the face, saying that he cannot stand him and that he has an opportunistic character. Nor does he speak with his parents.
- The father and mother work in the family business, and Marck has a "tempestuous" relationship with them. It seems that they forced him to enroll to study medicine, while Marck would have liked to work in the company.

In all this complexity, it is clear to the andrologist that touching Marck's body could in fact result in an explosion of anguish, insecurity, and anger.

Andrological surgery is an idea that Marck does not want to give up. However, he has agreed with the andrologist surgeon and psychosexologist to postpone the decision after working therapeutically on dysmorphism and the ideal of Schwarzenegger.

6.4 Conclusion

"Difficult patients" often present for complex andrological surgery, and this is worrying for the surgical and medical teams.

Clinical experience and the integrated andrologist-psychosexologist approach require an individualized clinical contract with a patient-friendly clinical and sexological preparatory path, with regard to both methods and timing.

Every adult and every teenager are like a world to be understood and perceived in both virtuous aspects and pathological behavior. The constant interaction with each individual regarding surgical techniques and possible prognosis, in the face of dysmorphism or psoriasis or mood deflection, gradually builds a clinical contract in which the patient is also responsible.

6.5 Sample Questionnaire for Anamnesis

Proposed by the psychosexologist to the patient (Marck).

1. You told me that you felt mocked by many doctors from childhood. Except by your psychiatrist, why should you trust us (andrologist and psychosexologist)?
2. If your parents were here, what would they tell me about your physicality?
3. When you think of Matilde, does it not bother you to know that she entertains other men?
4. If you had three wishes, which parts of your body would you change?
5. Have you ever fallen in love?
6. If your body were to remain what it is today, despite reaching 100 kg of lean mass, what do you think would happen in your life?
7. When you do the exercises in the gym and look at yourself in the mirror: what do you think? The other body builders, what will they think of your body?
8. What reassuring idea could lead you to trust a woman?

References

1. Jafferany M et al (2017) Evaluation of body parts that concern teenagers with body dysmorphic disorder. Prim Care Companion CNS Disord 19(5):154–159
2. Pope CG et al (2000) The Adonis complex. Simon & Schuster, New York
3. Nardomne G (2003) Al di là dell'amore e dell'odio per il cibo. Guarire rapidamente dalle patologie alimentari. BUR, Milano
4. Zappa LE (2009) Alice in fuga dallo specchio. Il disturbo dell'immagine corporea nell'anoressia nervosa e nei DCA. Franco Angeli, Milano
5. Cash TF et al (1990) Current and vestigial effects of overweight among women and men: fear of fat, attitudinal body, image and eating behaviors. J Psychopathol Behav Assess 12: 157–167

7 Body Image, Homosexuality, and Emotional Brain

In the homosexual experience, the body assumes very precise values: it is sculpted, muscular, smooth, athletic, and trim.

Numerous studies have shown higher levels of dissatisfaction in male homosexual patients than in heterosexual individuals [1].

Males with homosexual orientation seem more vulnerable than heterosexual males to eating disorders [2]: they pay greater attention to their choice of foods and to their weight, show a higher discrepancy between ideal physical fitness and the real body, and are more prone to depression and low self-esteem.

Clinical experience and 27 studies (a total of 5220 subjects) confirm that homosexual males, compared to heterosexuals, are characterized by an increased risk of developing pathological disorders associated with body image [3].

Consequently, homosexual patients (as do heterosexual women) consider a slender body an element of allure and ideal beauty; failure to achieve these objectives will result in shame, guilt, anger, and a propensity for an increasingly restricted diet.

7.1 Body Dissatisfaction and Food and Sexuality Disorders

Clinical research [2] indicates that 20% of males with eating disorders will have a homosexual orientation, while 42% (in a study of 156 patients) will have bulimic disorders.

In this respect, it would seem that homosexual individuals want to attract their partners by focusing on their physical attractiveness: slenderness, a young and toned body, wide shoulders, flat and defined abdomen, and sculpted biceps, focusing then on the physical appearance of the partner much more than in heterosexual couples.

This is not all.

To date, few studies have examined sexual satisfaction in single homosexuals and, in particular, the size of the penis as a cause of sexual dysfunction. The results

E. V. Longhi et al., *Psychosexual Counseling in Andrological Surgery*,
https://doi.org/10.1007/978-3-319-99646-2_7

would generally indicate a tendency to underestimate the size of one's member (26%), 17% would consider it "too small," and 12% would like to increase the length.

A study of 500 homosexual patients shows in particular that attitudes toward sexuality are conditioned by the perception of one's own genitality, in particular the penis and testicles.

In a hospital and surgical context, these characteristics can be highlighted by obsessive-compulsive behavior, repeated requests to surgeons for explanations, phobias toward clinical procedures, tension in the relationship with the medical team, and requests for reassurance about the outcome of the operation.

Summing up all these aspects, the literature has conceptualized two types of compulsiveness in homosexual patients: general and somatic.

The former would be associated with anxiety and sadness linked to the perception of possible criticism and external judgments toward one's own body image (considered liable to attack and lacking attractiveness); the latter would be derived from dissatisfaction with one's physical appearance, which is considered inadequate and weak, compared to ideal canons of beauty, and is consequently "under surgical attack."

It is not difficult to highlight a series of feelings and behaviors, directed toward the outside world and, in particular, the medical team (in a clinical context) which derive from a presumed dissatisfaction with the body:

1. Aggression
2. Avoidance
3. Masking
4. Destructiveness
5. Compensation
6. Pride and social compensation
7. Pride and rebellion

7.1.1 Aggression

This refers to defensive and oppositional attitudes in situations considered a hazard (pre-anesthesia with phobia of needles and cannulae) or in angry behavior toward those who may show criticism of gay sexual orientation and body image.

7.1.2 Avoidance

Another way to deal with situations that can cause shame: undressing in front of a doctor or a nurse, and more generally avoiding places of physical confrontation (gyms, swimming pools or mirrors) evidence disorders of a dysmorphobic type.

7.1.3 Masking

This is a way of dealing with shame and fear in the face of external confrontation. It conceals a body that is considered unsatisfactory with loose and concealing clothing; it uses cosmetics to reduce wrinkles and extends to surgical operations with prostheses to increase certain muscle groups (e.g., the calves) or to increase the volume of the member.

7.1.4 Destructiveness

A sort of self-directed aggression, induced, for example, by a nonideal body weight, which injures the individual with harmful practices: very rigid diets, physical exercise several times a day, and surgical procedures to reduce fat.

7.1.5 Compensation

An excessive regimen of body care to avoid loneliness, affective abandonment, disapproval, and lack of seductiveness. Thus, shaping the chest and biceps in the gym and wearing aggressive clothing become a means of countering low self-esteem, depression, and emotional fragility.

7.1.6 Pride and Social Compensation

Some patients show an excessive pride in achieving social success and admiration. They try to outdo other individuals in physical attractiveness and in having a multifaceted culture and a relaxed sexuality in order to feel admired, desired as partners, and strengthened in self-esteem.

7.1.7 Pride and Rebellion

To combat social prejudices and possible criticism of identity and sexual orientation, some patients behave like prima donnas, railing against any provocation or presumed criticism of their appearance and behavior. They rebel to increase their self-esteem, in a permanent climate of resistance, against everything and everyone, even doctors. Any clinical suggestion that may interfere with the patient's decision to undergo surgery, often invasive, is met with hysterical aggressiveness and rebellion.

When this defensive control is successful, it gives rise to pride and a sense of superiority that can be expressed as a competition with the medical team and a challenge to the psychosexologist "come on, let's see how good you are…."

As Goss and Gilbert [4] show, the considerable stress of these patients and the precariousness of the homosexual body image place important emotional pressures on the psychosexologist and doctors.

Clinical experience has taught us to avoid the challenge inherent in these behaviors, which conceal shame, fear of failure, anxiety, and anger.

The psychosexologist is the first figure to confront them:

> *I can see that you are very good at challenging and I thank you for having shown me this. I know you are telling me important things but I have to admit that I do not respond well to the language of challenge. I'm counting on your patience to translate them into another communication model...and I know I can count on your commitment....*

Ultimately, only a proper understanding of personal identity and homosexual body image can contribute to an understanding of the patient's issues, family and nonfamily relationships, expectations regarding the surgeon, the operation itself, and his current sex life.

Last but not least, the gender of the psychosexologist should not be underestimated in relation to the therapeutic contract and the relationship with doctors. When asked directly:

> *If rather than being a woman...I were a man...how would your feelings change?*

some patients respond that they feel more comfortable talking to a woman because a male therapist would compete with them with regard to virility and sexual performance.

But underlying this statement, there is always a hint that the patient is flattering to deceive, to be welcomed, to seduce in some way, and to overcome the shame of.

<living against the tide (Stephan, 21 years old) where even if you like, you must always show everyone that you are up to the situation and then .... in the evening you stay alone with yourself>

These broad reflections must, however, be seen in the context of the patient's growth path and the identification of sexual orientation.

There are four types of homosexuality:

1. Random: Transient experience.
2. Situated: Determined by context needs (e.g., prisons).
3. Personalized: Undeclared homosexuality.
4. Lifestyle: "Declared" homosexuals. In this, one should ask oneself: How much is declared? And to whom?

7.2 Homosexual Children and Their Parents

At what point in the life of an adolescent or a man does an andrological diagnosis and subsequent surgery take place? Sometimes, it is right alongside the revelation of homosexuality to one's parents or confession to them in the hospital context or, again, not far from it but in an emotional climate still in the making, for both children and parents.

A really painful experience for the patient, but even more serious for the parents, who are pervaded by feelings of anger, embarrassment, rejection and guilt. This can lead to extreme reactions such as the exclusion of the son from the family system.

In these cases, the psychosexologist can help parents to face the shock, to overcome the crisis, and to understand the process of outing that they are going through. Of course, the surgical procedure is postponed until the patient and the family have reached a new psychic balance.

Why wait for precisely that moment? The reasons are many and personal.

Case History

"You must be number one," my parents always tell me (Robert, 16 years old), but when they heard about the circumcision, I saw they were disoriented. For them, being real men is important. My mother lost her father at 8 years of age, and having a son was a blessing, she says. I do not feel I can keep it secret. My maternal grandmother realized when I was 9 years old. She simply said to me: "bring your friends back here as well, it would please me. We'll tell your parents later…." And I did. A catastrophe: my mother has not spoken to me for a week, and my father showed me all his disapproval. "Couldn't you have kept it to yourself? It knocked me back…."

Despite the high probability of disapproval, studies show that 60–77% of homosexuals decide to declare themselves to their parents in order to bring them closer together and to have a relationship based on honesty [5].

Conversely, leaving parents in the dark leads homosexual patients to avoid long-term sexual relationships or to introduce a female friend to relatives, in order to allude to a possible heterosexual relationship that soothes their anxieties [6].

Parents sometimes, although suspicious, prefer to downplay other possibilities of relationship in order to avoid admitting the homosexuality of their son. In the medical context, many parents think that they can "heal" the patient around the time of an operation, taking advantage of "medical and sexual knowledge."

It is true that at the moment of revelation, families are overwhelmed by a "powerful emotional wave" [7] that leads them to accuse their son of selfishness and to intimidate him to "change his mind, to restore the family balance once and for all."

Taken to extremes:

> I have been living with my mother since my parents separated 10 years ago (Rudolf, 22 years old). I often saw my father who suspected that I was gay and who ended up punching me during a football game, so that I would go back to 'being a man.' From that moment on, I refused to see him. I told my mother that I was homosexual and she wept. I have experienced mood swings since then and I have a sense of guilt for all the moments I haven't shared with my father…. I haven't seen him for 5 years. Today, I have to have the operation, I am afraid. I wish he was here….

From a psychosexological point of view, it would be a mistake to attribute responsibility for the negative reaction of parents entirely to them or to the culture to which they belong.

Often children self-reveal themselves during a quarrel or a discussion, and even the healthiest family can enter into a crisis of values and "go to pieces" losing its identity and, in time, family structure.

In approaching traumatized families, Guerin and Pendagast [8] recommend that psychosexologists and therapists, in general, help individuals express their feelings in a way that calms their souls and gives vent to their emotionality.

To then, take into account the needs and requirements of parents and child.

7.3 Acceptance

Most mothers and fathers assume that their children will grow up heterosexually, and when they are faced with the "difference," they feel a deep sense of failure [9]: both personal and in relation to future projects.

Five stages through which parents must pass to reach a state of acceptance of reality [10]:

1. Shock
2. Denial
3. Sadness and anger
4. Depression
5. Acceptance of the son's sexual orientation

Research shows that parents' attitudes toward their child's homosexuality can improve over time, because they gradually manage to rework the pain and make the sense of belonging to the family prevail.

After all, the children themselves have high hopes of acceptance from their parents, but they do not always manage to observe family reactions as stages in an ongoing process, just as was the path of accepting their homosexuality for them.

If they perceive the pain and anger of their parents as part of a temporary process, they can avoid symmetrical reactions of defense and strong aversion to them, which would naturally lead them to avoidance and emotional distancing.

It is however possible that some parents will not be able to have a smooth relationship with their homosexual children with the same willingness and empathy as before the revelation.

Moreover, in a hospital surgical context, the psychosexologist, having outlined the general and affective needs of the child and the parents, can offer a first containment, work on the strongest reactions, and program a "therapeutic work in progress," before surgery, although not without discussion with the medical surgical team, the patient, and the family in a project for which they are jointly responsible with regard to timing and manner.

Clinical Sample

"My partner Frank (Manuel, 25) accompanied me to the hospital. My father will come tomorrow. He is abroad for work and my mother doesn't like Frank. She will come tonight. I feel that I have disappointed her, that I have added pain to pain."

"What do you mean?" (psychosexologist)

"My brother Erick died aged 8, of brain neoplasia. Four years of disease, surgery and radiotherapy. My mother just crumbled and my father threw himself into his work. I was 15 years old at the time. I have always studied, done my best in school and in sport, so as not to give them problems, they took me to a therapist while I was facing up to the death of my brother and right there I realized my sexual orientation. I felt alone and I kept the secret to myself."

"do you think that your parents would not be willing to talk about it today? If you want, we can do it together… in any case, I need information from them. Your future, your relationship cannot be conditioned by these silences. Passive suffering does not allow you and them to build with serenity. Then we'll also talk to Frank. One step at a time.... The doctors and the surgeon, are waiting for information from us." (psychosexologist)

7.4 Mind Psyche and Emotions

Thus far, the psyche, sexuality, and the systemic therapeutic approach. It would however be a mistake to neglect neuroscience and the emotional brain. Biologically oriented neuropsychiatry has shown the links between pathological or disturbed behavior and brain structures.

When the psychosexologist comes face to face with an andrological patient, waiting for surgery, he/she must also refer to the role of the limbic system and the limbic-encephalic structures.

In this specific case, recognizing a dysmorphic, narcissistic, borderline disorder, for example, means appreciating the clinical and symptomatological characteristics.

According to Marsel Mesalum [11], various brain zones can be distinguished, each with poorly defined boundaries but with specific neuro-functional and behavioral characteristics. The human brain therefore seems to be characterized by parallel and simple information processing.

It seems that the human brain has three essential competences:

1. To connect with the outside world through the sensory brain system
2. To produce response behaviors (motor, emotional, behavioral, attentive linguistics, etc.)

3. Internally to elaborate data before providing answers, the most elaborate and complex activity, in dysmorphic disorder, narcissism, pathological relational behavior, and eating disorders

There are five functional zones of the cerebral cortex, and each of these zones has a neuronal heritage with differentiated competences in respect to others:

1. **Primary**, motor sensory.
2. **Unimodal associative** which allows for an initial processing of data, for example, acoustic, visual, tactile, olfactory, and taste data.
3. **Associative heteromodal** where information is processed in a more complex and integrated way. There are *three* distinct brain areas: one posterior (at the posterior parietal cortex); one inferior, important for integrating visual, linguistic, and emotional stimuli; and one anterior, the most extensive and the most evolved (prefrontal cortex) which distinguishes human from animal behavior, highly emotional.
4. **Paralimbic** which interfaces the various cognitive processes and which analyses the information, regulating priority, the congruity of the answers, and sequentiality.
5. **Limbic** which regulates in a specific way the needs and drives and which originates the "innate" behaviors of the individual.

The limbic system in particular comprises various interconnected structures and provides emotional and motivational meanings to our existence.

There are primary emotions, such as anger, fear, panic, sadness, surprise, disgust, and simple emotions not mediated by other complex functional areas that give rise to instinctive reactions.

These are followed by more complex emotions, linked to social behavior, which seem to respond to two distinct needs:

1. Gaining approval, not disappointing the expectations of others
2. Conquering affection, love, and admiration

These emotions of the second type are called social. Social emotions can have a negative or a positive value.

The right brain hemisphere regulates our primary emotions to almost exclusively negative value, whereas the left brain hemisphere regulates the emotionality, the intrapsychic stimuli to positive value.

Only at the beginning of 2000, we did begin to speak of emotional intelligence [12] to describe the ability to read, interpret, and respond appropriately to the feelings, needs, and behaviors of others, using one's emotions in an appropriate way to motivate, plan, and achieve health, sex, and quality of life objectives.

Emotional intelligence (EQ/EI) is therefore a crucial element in the regulation of emotional activity, through the control of impulses and electrophysiological responses: heartbeat, sweat, tears, etc.

An understanding of neuroscience and neuropsychiatry makes the psychosexologist not just a psychologist with wider clinical knowledge but a clinician with more a specific training that facilitates the diagnostic, surgical, and rehabilitation process alongside doctors and surgeons, leaving them the priority role and contract with the patient.

All the while, playing a role of comparison, investigation, and evaluation with the individual patient, his history, family, reference systems (school, work, etc.), and the surgical context that will accompany him in a new process of health, aesthetics, and pleasure.

7.5 Conclusion

Homosexual orientation does not have univocal and comparable somatic characteristics and ethics. Clinical research has shown significant pathological variables on the identity of the body image. However, we must not generalize, lest we fall into classifications and generalizations inappropriate to the process of individual health. Psychiatric, psychological, systemic, and neuropsychological knowledge can help to highlight the strengths and weaknesses of each individual, assessing a low level of emotional and clinical risk in any planned surgery. Working in a team means creating a fluid and co-responsible complexity, respecting the psychic and physical balance of each individual patient, of whatever sexual orientation.

References

1. Hoffmann S et al (2018) Patterns of body image concerns in adolescence and early adulthood: a latent profile analysis. Eat Behav 29:28–34
2. Woityna E et al (2017) Gender, body image and social support: biopsychosocial determinants of depression among patients with psoriasis. Acta Derm Venereol 97(1):91–97
3. Suen YT (2017) Body talk of single homosexuals: resist and keep the discourse on ageing in the gay community. J Homosex 64(3):397–414
4. Goss K, Gilbert P (2002) Eating disorders, shame and pride. A cognitive behavioural functional analysis. In: Gilbert P et al (eds) Body shame. Brunner-Routledge, East Sussex, pp 219–255
5. LaSala M (2000) Homosexuals and their parents: family therapy for seizures following the revelation of his homosexuality. Fam Process 39:1
6. Harry J (1988) Some problems of gay/lesbian families. In: Chilman C et al (eds) Variant family forms: families in trouble series, vol 5. Sage, Newbury Park, pp 96–113
7. Bowen M (1978) Family therapy in clinical practice. Jason Aronson, New York
8. Guerin P, Pendagast E (1976) Evaluation of family system and genogram. In: Guerin P (ed) Family therapy: theory and practice. Gardner Press, New York, pp 450–465
9. Muller A (1987) Parents matter: parent's relationships with lesbian daughters and gay son. The Naiad Press, Tallahassee
10. Robinson B et al (1989) Response of parents to learning that their child is homosexual and concern over AIDS: a national study. J Homosex 18:59–80

11. Mesulam MM (1990) Large scale neurocognitive networks and distributed processing of attention, language and memory. Ann Neurol 28:597–613
12. Ross ED et al (1994) Hemispheric lateralization of primary and social emotion implications for developing a comprehensive neurology for emotions, repression and the subconscious. Neuropsychiatry Neuropsychol Behav Neurol 7:1–19

8 The Doctor-Patient Relationship Referral to the Sexologist and How to Be Understood by Patients

Communicating with the patient is an art, a discipline, and a unique relationship. Every doctor, of course, has his/her own style, a nonverbal manner, and an effective interview technique. However, it needs not be generalized.

Every doctor is well suited to some patients who are particularly in tune with their character and personality. With other people it is difficult to establish a collaborative relationship, not because of inexperience but because of psychological and motivational characteristics which are different from their own.

To make communication smoother, we must always remember that the doctor-patient relationship depends on three variables: the context, the patient, and the doctor.

The relationship is conditioned by the place where the patient lives, the psychological makeup of the patient, the pathology he suffers from, the worry inherent in surgery, the ability of the doctor to welcome individuals, and the goal that the specialist sets.

The first consultation or the first doctor-patient assessment reveals different characteristics, depending on whether it takes place in a university health facility or in a private setting.

In the first case, the patient comes into contact with a situation mediated by administrative and nursing staff who, despite their best intentions, unwittingly create discomfort for the patient due to urgent outpatient care needs or delays in the performance of clinical examinations, perhaps accompanied by sharp replies or unclear directions.

In this context, clinical experience teaches the surgeon to ask the patient some introductory questions that allow him to be heard not only regarding his pathology but in relation to the individual.

Did you have difficulty parking? Maybe you found a long queue at Reception, I'm sorry you had to wait….

E. V. Longhi et al., *Psychosexual Counseling in Andrological Surgery*,
https://doi.org/10.1007/978-3-319-99646-2_8

Anachronistic? My professor of psychopathology taught me that a brief introductory chat, prior to an anamnestic review, albeit a recorded one, makes the first doctor-patient approach less formal.

On the other hand, taking the details of the disease quickly and concisely could cause dissatisfaction in the patient and perplexity about the diagnosis and the surgical course proposed.

In the private context, the patient presupposes being welcomed into a hospitable, de-pathologizing, non-anxiogenic environment and with a team of assistants who offer empathy and kindness to the individual.

Human contact is more instinctive and less forced in the context of the first visit during which the patient usually feels freer to express his or her concerns, symptoms, and emotionality, without having the anxiety of the time limit of a normal visit to a university facility.

Last but not least, the doctor-patient conversation is rarely interrupted by intrusions, not even necessary ones, by the nursing staff, often without knocking on the door. During the examination, the patient can undress in a private setting and may also be offered a tunic to make him feel at ease.

In any event, it is essential to observe the patient's attitude toward the disease and the possible surgery. That is, what does he think about his problem, if it worsens, becomes dramatic, or, conversely, diminishes? Whether he has already had other surgical experiences or is encountering his first surgery and whether his family history has been marked by a series of surgical interventions or so far, none of its members has had such experience.

8.1 Doctor-Patient Approaches

Since not all patients are the same, clinical experience teaches us to use an initial observational tactic in the doctor-patient interview, before identifying the type of patient.

Many studies have tried to synthesize models of the doctor-patient approach and the reactions of the patient in the face of a surgical prognosis.

From the concepts of Hollender, the American medical psychologist (see Table 8.1), to the criterion of the German physician Viktor Emil von Gebsattel (1883–1976) (see Table 8.2), where the doctor-patient relationship would be based on the concept of distance between the two individuals.

8.1.1 Determination of Patient Type

Models aside, clinical experience shows that the secret to the professional success of doctors, and surgeons in particular, has largely to do with the psychological and analytical abilities of the patient, some of whom are in fact already pathologically confronted with the possibility of surgery (Table 8.3).

Table 8.1 Doctor-patient relationship according to the Hollender model (1958)

Relationships according to the activeness/passiveness criterion. Similar situations in psycho-affective development
Activeness of the doctor-passiveness of the patient
Patient is completely passive; the doctor is the sole manager of decisions. Conditions: coma, myocardial infarction, stroke, and surgery under general anesthesia. Also with mental confusion, deterioration, and psychiatric imbalances. To implement the therapeutic intervention, the doctor acts with decisional and operational autonomy, and the patient must let him/her do so. In psycho-affective development, the prototype is represented by the mother-neonatal (dependent) relationship
Doctor direction-patient compliance
The patient collaborates with the doctor in implementing the therapy prescribed by the doctor. The patient is aware of his condition and of the usefulness of therapy. Conditions: infectious diseases, dysendocrinism, vascular not serious, and all and acute situations in which the patient is able to collaborate. Prototype in psycho-affective development: childhood, in which the child follows the teachings of parents who guide the process of autonomy
Reciprocal doctor-patient collaboration
The healthcare professional is occasionally consulted to obtain information on the progress of the disease and to change the treatment. Conditions: rehabilitation therapy, psychotherapy, in chronic diseases; diabetes, cardiovascular pathologies, senility disorders, psychic disorders in psychotherapy. Prototype: relationship of two mature adults

Table 8.2 Von Gebsattel model

First phase	*Human appeal*	The doctor immediately responds to the request for help and declares his unconditional availability
Second phase	*Distancing*	The patient is subjected to clinical examinations and is considered an "object of study" and no longer in the emotional relationship
Third phase	*Personalization*	The patient is emotionally reconciled and involved with the diagnostic, surgical, and healing phases

Table 8.3 Pathological ways of facing surgical intervention

• Patients who refuse a necessary operation: they do not see the point of the operation or use "denial" or have experienced pain (in infancy) in this field
• Patients who request unnecessary operations: subjects with masochistic tendencies or with remedial needs (guilt) or with psychotic disorders

Understanding the question and the correct relationship with the patient allows:

(a) Processing of latent conflicts
(b) Therapeutic response to the body and mind

There is however no doubt that the most common reason for dissatisfaction on the part of the patient is the lack of detailed explanations by the doctor regarding the pathology, surgical intervention, the length of stay, discharge, and post-surgical care.

Every surgeon of course tries to use every communicative tool in order to be clear, explicit, reassuring, and accommodating. However, the patient listens through the anxiety of not understanding, the anxiety of the unexpected operation, and the anxiety of the absence from work, of the family balance, and the sense of emptiness of "no longer feeling like the man he was before."

This means arranging for a series of colleagues to reiterate, in a different way, what the surgeon has already described, perhaps more than once.

Talking with the anesthetist is an important opportunity to quell doubts about the side effects of sedation, any allergies to pharmacological substances the patient may have, the treatments taken and which might need to be suspended a few days before the operation, anxiety over "non-recovery," and any depressive, anxiety-producing aspects of the patient's character.

Not forgetting that the patient's psychological investment will also be conditioned by the type and extent of the intervention. With reference to the genital area, it is unquestionable that the patient will alternate latent sensations of hypothetical castration with anxiety about the aesthetic and sexual outcomes of surgery.

It is not by chance that the study by Dr. Wendy Levinson [1], published in the JAMA (*The Journal of the American Medical Association*), states that:

> "Effective communication makes the client more satisfied and brings better results in terms of health recovery" and further that "patients decide to sue the doctor (surgeon) who treated them, not for 'incompetence or professional negligence' but for the way in which he treated them at an interpersonal level." Thus "ineffective communication leads to side effects, poor therapeutic compliance and, in the absence of appreciable results, patient dissatisfaction."

In a study similar to that of Dr. Levinson's, Dr. G.R. Hickson found that doctors who had never been reported as being ill at work were described by patients as "communicative people, more inclined to participate emotionally in the evolution of health in pre- and post-surgery and more willing to be contacted by patients and to come into contact with them."

Finally, as Peter Maguire and Carolyn Pitceathly claim in an article published in the *British Medical Journal* in 2002, "When doctors use communication skills effectively, both they and patients benefit" (Table 8.4).

8.1.2 The Time Factor

Despite the good intentions of many surgeons to communicate effectively with the patient, the time available seems to be a very limited variable in university facilities.

Table 8.4 Benefits of effective communication [2]

1. Doctors very precisely identify the patients' problems
2. Patients are more satisfied with the way they are followed and can better understand their problems, diagnostic examinations, surgical treatments, and the post-surgical phases in hospital and on discharge
3. Patients are more likely to adhere to treatment and follow advice about behavioral changes
4. Anxiety and predisposition to anxiety and depression decrease
5. The doctor himself benefits and works better

According to the results of a study by Langewitz and colleagues, published in the *British Medical Journal* in 2002:

1. The doctor stops the patient's account of his symptoms about 22 s after the beginning.
2. Ninety percent of patients spontaneously finish the story within 92 s and all within 2 min.
3. In the space between 22 and 92 s, 75% of symptoms are mentioned. In other words, the more the patient describes his symptoms in detail, the more he remembers interesting details to the benefit of a comprehensive understanding of the problem.

There is more. To these figures can be added other data, backed up by detailed studies on doctor-patient communication:

1. Thirty-six percent of patients do not remember the information provided by the doctor regarding prognosis and surgery [3].
2. Seventy percent of patients incorrectly take in information about drugs to be discontinued and/or to be continued in reduced doses before surgery [3].
3. Doctors generally underestimate the patient's desire for information in 65% of clinical interviews [4].
4. During a 20-min interview, little more than 60 s is devoted to the transmission of information to patients [4].

Clinical experience, however, trains us to observe other aspects of the patient: nonverbal communication and emotions, even lies, reticence, signs of anxiety, and depression.

It is not by chance that Mehrabian [5] showed that physicians and patients, face to face, communicate only 7% through verbal messages; 38% through tone of voice, speed, or slowness of speech; and 55% through nonverbal communication: facial expressions, posture, direction of gaze, hand gestures, etc.

There is a great deal of information that might remain in the shadows due to the patient's modesty, his fear of receiving very bad news about his health, or his feeling of awe for the doctor. This information can be acquired by the surgeon through his ability to discern nonverbal communication (his own and that of the interlocutor), creating a climate of relaxation and openness to communicate confidence, accessibility, and collaboration with the patient.

This creates the conditions for an empathic and accommodating therapeutic path, in five steps:

1. Effective communication
2. Patient understanding and trust
3. Adhesion to the treatment (compliance)
4. Efficacy of the treatment
5. Patient satisfaction

8.1.3 Referral to the Psychosexologist

The therapeutic alliance is made up of many ingredients that have been treated in different ways in the previous chapters.

The patient is in a position to observe and to unconsciously monitor the feelings among the doctors (distrust, competition or communication skills, esteem, and affability) and to experience their charm or distrust.

In this context, referral to colleagues and in particular to the psychosexologist becomes a very delicate act in the surgical setting. Errors made in clinical experience have led to the discovery of more mechanisms of referral, some more effective and others unsuitable, dry, and scarcely empathic.

Initially a neutral style was considered:

> *It is our team's practice that you (the patient) meet some colleagues and among them the psychosexologist.*
>
> *Our team includes a psychosexologist.*

These and similar formulations, though delivered in good faith, overlooked the patient's feelings, which were soon made clear.

> I am not crazy…I have no psychological problems
>
> are you offloading me to your colleague? Will I see her in the operating room?

They carry the risk of creating anxiety about a figure whose role is not always clearly understood (the psychosexologist) and an opinion toward a patient (and partner) considered emotionally unsuitable for surgery, unless the opinion of the psychosexologist is otherwise.

Each patient has an individualized diagnostic procedure according to clinical characteristics, personality, and family structure.

In accordance with the characteristics of our team, surgeons today make a heartfelt invitation to the patient and partner:

> *…Now that we have outlined the stages of the surgical process and of the hospital stay, I would like to reassure you that even after being discharged you will not be alone. In this regard, I ask you to be patient enough to meet a colleague of mine (the psychosexologist) so that we can provide you with further information on how we can make you feel at your best during the stay, reassure your relatives and then accompany you in the post-surgical phase. Since surgery interferes with a delicate pelvic part of masculinity, we are concerned that your resumption of sexual activity be smooth and effective.…*

It is not perhaps the perfect referral, but it is one which follows a therapeutic contract, where the patient is at the center of attention and where doctors try from the very first approach to build an individualized clinical project, tailored to the character and sensitivity of the patient and to the sexual style of the couple.

In the meantime, the psychosexologist has already collated the clinical information regarding the patient and the recommendations for the surgical procedure, along with the first impressions of the surgeon.

At the first interview, it is important for me to go to meet the patient at the door of the clinic and to invite to the interview the patient's partner, if accompanied, or, in the case of an adolescent, the parents.

8.2 Children and Adolescents

In the latter scenario, to my question:

How do you see your child's situation?

parents describe their concern and the character traits of the boy:

he is shy and taciturn…he always speaks so little…he seems daunted by the operation…

and then compare this with the boy asking him:

Do you see yourself in your parents' description?

Then, having created a channel of communication, of availability, and of collaboration, I ask (the parents):

Could I have your permission to speak alone with Erick?

And of the boy:

Do you feel like talking to me?

The pace for me is dictated by the emotional nature of my interlocutors and by the need to give everyone a fair chance. If the child is a minor, I agree with the young patient on the topics to be referred to the parents, to allow them to participate in our therapeutic process. Once the parents are invited back to interview, the young patient is helped to relate the important points of the interview, so that he feels that he is the protagonist of his own health and intimacy.

I like to thank everyone for their availability and for the time they have given me: no less than 60 min. I can say that I have more information to give to the surgeon and that I will write up my notes and send them to him by e-mail. Patient and parents will receive the same notes by c/c.

In this way, the psychosexologist shows him/herself to be a facilitator of communication:

1. Within the medical team
2. Between the patient and the surgeon
3. Between the family, the patient, the surgeon, and the medical team

The approach with an adult patient and partner is different.

8.3 Adults

The adult patient is welcomed in the same way, but I immediately thank the partner for having accepted the surgeon's invitation:

> *if your partner is available, tell her to accompany you on a visit to my colleague the psychosexologist.*

and the patient for the availability he has given me and the medical team.

In Mediterranean culture, the partner has an unwitting therapeutic role. It is she who chooses the surgeon she relies on, the hospital, and whom she trusts among doctors. She assesses how much the team can cope with the situation in the pre- and post-surgery phases.

They are initially asked:

> *How do you see the situation? The surgeon told me that you have agreed on the surgical process and discussed many delicate parts of the preparation for the operation.*

Why this prologue? The surgeon, no matter how empathic and helpful he may be, cannot build an equal relationship with the patient: he has a surgical and clinical responsibility.

But in compliance and in the sexual recovery after discharge, the patient and partner are the protagonists of their lives, and from the beginning, as a psychosexologist, I make this explicit.

Moreover, meeting the couple also means understanding the moment in their lives when the surgical diagnosis crept in, interrupting projects, opportunities, and desires.

Case 1
"We have been living together for 2 years," reports Mary, 32. "He (the partner) had a previous marriage from which he has two children, now teenagers. This is my second long term cohabitation… There is an 18 year difference between us and we were trying for a child when this happened to us (surgery)…."

Case 2
"We have known each other for 4 years and we still don't live together," recounts Albert, 43. "We are looking for a house and we would like to get married in a year's time. She (the partner) is very afraid because she suffers from endometriosis and fears that she cannot give me a child."

Case 3

"I'm scared," says Sylvie, 38, "it seems to me that everything happens to me. A month ago, my gynaecologist told me that I had started the menopause (early) and now him, (the partner) with a diagnosis of neoplasm in the penis...."

Case 4

"We have two twins, through artificial insemination" explains Julius, 48. "We had them late and my partner feels like half a mother. She's depressed and it's not the same anymore...She's put on 10 kg in the last year... and now my situation has depressed her even more. I don't know what to do...."

Once accepted and shared, the revelations of the couple can become the keystone for understanding, for each patient and for each partner, whose nonclinical meanings the surgery takes on and whose nonsexual meanings have their own intimacy, as a vehicle to reopen themselves to future projects and to have the possibility of success and continuity of the future, like other couples.

What does this mean for surgeons? The main data. The information is discussed by the team and the communication style which will ease and lessen the emotionality of the patient and the partner is postulated. My presence is planned during hospitalization, in conversation with the patient's partner. The first post-surgical interview with the psychosexologist will be held to compare the anxieties of the first interview with the outcome of the operation and to make sexuality an occasion for daily encounters with play and fantasy.

Who then is the psychosexologist? A specialist with a strong contract with the medical team, a short-term contract with the patient and partner, and an intense scientific and emotional contract with him/herself, not just a psychologist but a therapist, a sexologist, a post-surgical rehabilitator, a colleague to whom we owe nothing, except the ability to support the individuals and to draw the best qualities from them at a critical moment in the clinical process.

8.4 Conclusions

Doctor-patient communication is in itself a therapeutic step that no surgeon and no patient can renounce. Together they can connect clinical and interpersonal information in a quantity and of a quality, which is useful when defining the diagnosis, prognosis, and quality of life of the patient. Together they reduce the possibility of error, transfer the feeling of being included and welcomed as a patient and as a person, offer the patient professional and responsible care, and build a mutual relationship of esteem and trust.

8.5 Sample Self-Assessment for Communication Style Evaluation

This is not a test and no structured answers are expected. These are just a few questions that can make every specialist reflect on his or her own communicative style, posture, internal thoughts, and nonverbal communication.

A kind of self-learning:

1. What do you feel before meeting a patient? (e.g., do you want to make a good impression, amaze them with your professionalism…?)
2. How do you think the patient judges your approach? (e.g., empathic, scientific, sterile…)
3. When you talk to the patient, where do you look? (e.g., at the anamnesis folder to be filled in, at the ground, at the partner…)
4. When you have built a channel of communication with the patient, how have you gestured? (e.g., mixed, I always move my hands, play with the ballpoint…)
5. If the patient does not understand and asks you to repeat more clearly, what could be your first emotional reaction? (e.g., apologize, feel annoyed and intolerant, think he is a tough patient…)
6. When you explain the surgery to the patient, what means do you use? (e.g., photographs, a quick sketch, the computer…)
7. What do you think a patient would not forgive you? (e.g., haste, impatience, poor dialogue…)
8. What kind of language do you prefer during the interview? (e.g., suitable for patient culture, understandable, scientific…)
9. If the patient presents himself for interview with a relative or partner, what is your first thought? (e.g., what do they want?, why are they interfering?, let's see what useful information they bring me…)
10. When you want to reassure a particularly anxious patient, how do you proceed? (e.g., reassuring arguments, physical contact, composure, asking relatives for help)
11. When you compare yourself with your colleagues and in particular with the psychosexologist, what do you think? (e.g., they give you useful information, they support you, they are another problem…)
12. What could be the distinctive quality that one of your patients could perceive at the time of discharge? (e.g., personal availability, my look, professional training…)
13. When a patient returns to the clinic after discharge, what do you hope? (e.g., that everything is fine, that they do not complain, that they don't take up too much time, that they come alone…)

References

1. Lewinson W (1997) Physician-patient communication: the relationship with malpractice claims among primary care physicians and surgeons. J Am Med Assoc 277(7):553–559
2. Maguire P, Pitceathly C (2002) The magical number seven, plus or minus two: some limits on our capacity to process information. Psychol Rev 63:81–97
3. Ley P (1979) Memory for medical information. Br J Clin Psychol 18(2):245–255
4. Waitzkin H (1984) Doctor-patient communication. Clinical implications of social scientific research. J Am Med Assoc 252(17):2441–2446
5. Mehrabian A (1972) Nonverbal communication. Aldine Publishing, Chicago

9 Sexological Anamnesis: How to Discover the Reasons for HIS and HER Intimacy

Observing an andrological patient, and in particular a patient presenting for surgery, requires well-defined methods and areas of investigation.

Unlike clinical diagnosis, sexological anamnesis frames the patient within the various reference systems, personal, cultural, geographical, political, and economic, and, not least, in the personal history, the relationship with his body, the relationship with partners, sexual education, and the relationship with the current partner if he describes a fixed relationship of at least a year (Fig. 9.1).

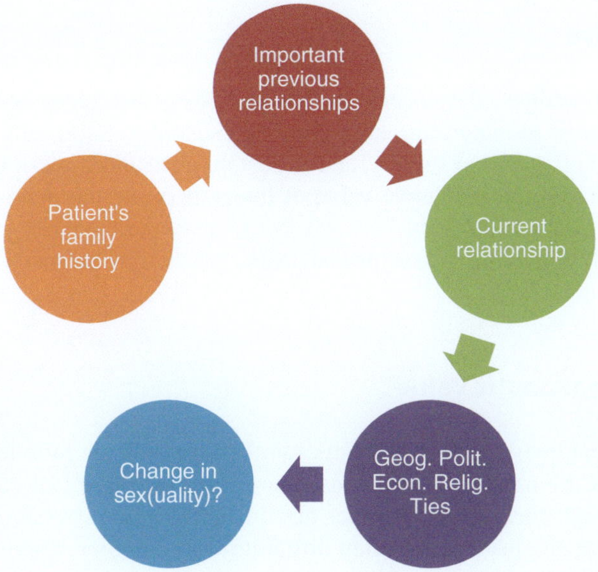

Fig. 9.1 Sexological anamnesis frames the patient within the various reference systems

E. V. Longhi et al., *Psychosexual Counseling in Andrological Surgery*,
https://doi.org/10.1007/978-3-319-99646-2_9

Table 9.1 Nine areas of sexological evaluation of the patient and the couple

• Personality and sensitivity of the patient
• Codification of relationships (previous partner, family of origin, friends, etc.) that they have best understood
• Body map awareness
• Quality of life of the individual
• Quality of life of the couple
• Quality of life in the family of origin
• View of the future
• Expectations of the doctor-patient relationship
• Expectations of the sexologist-patient relationship

Why? First of all, the characteristics are different from one man to the next, for example, those who live and work in a big city, where their masculinity is also insinuated by their professional career, their economic status, their qualifications, and their family authority, give great significance to physical and sexual performance even within the couple, a performance within the performance.

On the other hand, a man who lives in a less competitive environment, with a more normal life where his role is based on family enlargement and a non-stressful and hobby-rich decent standard of living, will confer on the sexuality of the couple a greater procreative value and could often confuse virility with fertility (Table 9.1).

9.1 Andrology and Sexology Integration

9.1.1 Above

In presurgical settings, the American Cancer Society has recently reaffirmed its pragmatic interest in integrating andrology and sexology: especially in the anamnestic phase, preparatory to surgery, and in post-surgical andro-sexological rehabilitation. Underlining the predictive value of integration and the most compromised areas (Table 9.2).

Therefore sexology possesses propaedeutic, predictive, perspective, and therapeutic value.

9.1.2 Propaedeutic Value

The sexological question always refers to other areas of the individual's and the partner's lives. Being able to hypothesize a priori how these factors will become complex through the surgical impact and in the following rehabilitation phase could prevent scenarios that are often difficult for the surgeon when managing the patient:

Table 9.2 Andro-sexological integration

Predictive value
In the presurgical phase, with the use of a neuro-sexological atlas, it is possible:
• To hypothesize the emotional impact on the patient of the surgery and his or her post-surgical compliance
• To lower anxiety about anesthesia
• To assess the role of the partner in the life of the patient
• To support a priori dealing with the discomfort of the change in continence and sexuality in the post-surgical phase
• To relieve the surgeon of emotional and relational encroachments that he cannot take on but to have the confidence of recognizing them and limiting their evolution
The most compromised areas:
• Intrapsychic (anxiety, depression, inadequacy, apathy, aggressive irritability)
• Sexual response
• Socialization and relations with the outside world
• Food-sleep
• Lifestyle with the partner

Phantom pains, burnout in taking sex pharmacotherapy, phobias, eating disorders, and drunkenness

Painful orgasm (other than DE) and drop in desire (depression from retrograde ejaculation)

9.1.3 Predictive and Perspective Value

Sexological anamnesis prior to surgery allows one to consider whether the patient has already had any phenomena of premature ejaculation, erectile dysfunction, and painful or delayed ejaculation or has been the victim of trauma. This has a considerable impact on any andrological and urological therapies, both in their evaluation and in their possible effects.

9.1.4 Therapeutic or Iatrogenic Value of the Partner

The sexuality of the partner. The change in sexual habits due to surgery also affects the sexual response of the partner.

Why? Sexuality in pre-surgery can reveal sexual dysfunction in the partner: anorgasmia, vaginismus, painful orgasm, postcoital cystitis, etc. The patient's concern will therefore be directed not only to the surgical intervention but also to hiding the sexual discomfort of the partner "to protect her." Hence, each half of the couple will try to restore the previous balance even at the expense of prescribed therapies or desired post-surgical results.

In practice:

Pre-surgical phase:

- Identification of the communication style to be followed between medical team and patient, to improve the compliance of the subject
- Anxiety management
- Redefinition of patient's doubts about post-surgery
- Guiding the patient through the surgical process
- Guiding the partner through the pre- and post-surgical process
- Variant: healthy partner or partner with previous gynecological and/or oncological surgical experience—mourning abortions

Primary post-surgical phase:

- Analysis of the emotional response of the patient and partner to the post-op symptoms
- Recomposition of emotional state and changes in quality of life of the patient and partner
- Comparison of differences in habits and emotionality of partners
- Individualized psychosexual rehabilitation intervention:
  - Scheduling of sexological exercises for the couple and for each individual partner
  - Recommendations for redefining anxio-depressive aspects, addiction, and phobias
- Team coordination of pharmachological, andrological, and sexological rehabilitation protocols
- Monitoring and prevention of burnout
- Supplementary sessions with the partner to prevent and or contain therapeutic sabotage

The literature [1] shows, among other things:

- Post-surgery, 63% of partners complain about him
- Adaptation dysfunction in the process of sexual and relational change of the couple
- Pre-existing anorgasmia masked by a reticent and reserved intimacy
- Changes in orgasm as a result of negative pre-marriage sexual experiences
- Changes in desire due to hidden marital conflicts

For example, in a patient who has received a penile prosthesis, sexual rehabilitation requires an individualized sex procedure, in particular in the achievement of:

- Erotic pleasure with erection
- Erection without orgasm
- Extravaginal orgasm
- Introduction of the penis into the vagina
- Coitus

9.2 Clinical Research also in the Anamnestic Phase

These are questionnaires that patients can more easily fill in, during anamnesis and, separately, at the end of the first interview. A sort of further verification of the data collected in the direct interview:

- Crown and Crisp Experiential Index (CCEI) for the psychological assessment of the current traumatic state
- Dyadic Adjustment Scale (DAS) quality of the relationship of the couple and the influence of same on:
  The progress of the pathology of the patient
  The compliance of the patient
- Aggression Questionnaire (AQ) for the evaluation of free anxiety, phobia, O.C.D., somatic symptoms, emotional decontrol, and depression
- Index of Sexual Satisfaction (ISS) for evaluation of the quality of intimacy of the couple and the impact of the patient's pathology on the "family body"

9.2.1 Psychosexologist, Male or Female?

In a mostly male urological and andrological team, the presence of a female psychosexologist is experienced by the patient as reassuring and not invasive of his sexuality because, in line with the patient's prejudice, a female psychosexologist has a language that will be understood and accepted by the partner.

The patient can feel protected and accepted, even in moments of aggression and anger, and the rehabilitation is experienced as "the general test" of one's own way of being, before facing the partner. A female therapist can enhance the feeling of being empathetically protected, while a male specialist medic can scientifically reconfirm the patient's virility.

This renders the patient free to say "goodbye" to the therapist and to forget her without guilt, and this renders the partner, who from the first meeting with the psychosexologist is defined as a "co-therapist," more involved and not just a tool at the service of the partner. Her wants, needs, and concerns will be considered with the same degree of attention during the post-surgical care of the patient.

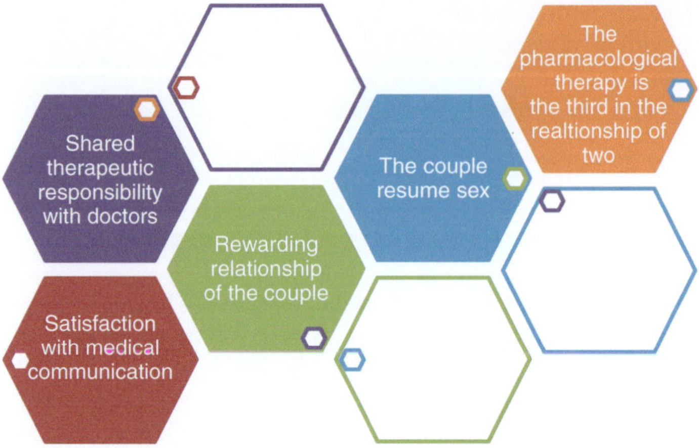

Fig. 9.2 Personal efficacy

Moreover, an essential element, the sexological rehabilitation exercises, will be defined by the needs of both partners, in terms of pleasure, play, fantasy, and the relational style of the couple.

Such was our team, chosen for its psycho-relational and clinical characteristics. Each team must be chosen according to its own model of approach toward the patient and to the partner.

Throughout all of this, any pharmacological prescription written by the andrologist on discharge should not be forgotten. It is not a simple oral prescription, especially if it is preparatory to the sexuality of the two. For the couple it is "a third" that conditions the partners' spontaneity and could exacerbate his sense of inadequacy and her lack of allure.

Also, during this transition, the psychosexologist justifies the therapeutic prescription as an added value to the intensity of the couple's relationship and a temporary controlling shareholder, to facilitate the partners in the recovery of sexuality.

The personal efficacy is shown in Fig. 9.2.

9.3 What Happens When Post-surgery Symptoms Disappear and Sexuality Resumes?

Normally the patient and partner report an initial sense of relief and pleasure in the patient with erectile dysfunction, followed by some anxiety and depression as soon as the male sexual response is "restored."

The partner may have an even more intense emotional response to the sudden new sexual potency of the partner: initial happiness with the sexual improvement of the partner with conduct and testimony of a positive responsiveness. This is followed (especially in the presence of conflict within the couple) by a series of hindering behaviors from the partner, which are aimed at stopping the therapy from proceeding, for example, decreased desire, psychosomatic symptoms (dermatitis, itching, tickling, anhedonia—lack of pleasure), and above all a complacent and at the same time competitive and symmetrical ambivalent relationship.

For some women, the partner may become "too powerful" and eager to engage with other partners, "too egocentric and competitive," "too seductive and greedy for female conquest"....

The psychosexologist often warns the couple in the presurgical phase about the emergence of impatience and behavior within the couple, which, if neglected, could condition the outcome of the intervention and therapeutic compliance.

"(partner) I had a miscarriage and I still feel anguish and guilt. I was very keen on it and he (the patient) only told me 'to be patient'...but now that he has to be operated on, it is me who has to understand, he told me, because he is afraid".

"(patient) I have always suffered because of my curved penis and now I have decided. I want to be normal...July (the partner) tells me that I'm obsessed, that I do it only for aesthetics...but then she complains if I don't look for her often enough".

In this emotional complexity, the psychosexologist acts with a systemic approach: he shows the couple that each is trying to be welcomed by the other and that anger and resentment now need to be addressed in a more constructive way.

Also because the outcomes of post-traumatic neurological and surgical stress after surgery will put them to the test, limiting their ability to filter feelings. Is this due to excessive production of cortisol? Not always. But clinical experience shows that the "depathologization of the couple" entails for both partners a sense of "absolution" and further encouragement in their mutual relational abilities.

This entails a therapeutic method through which the couple go over their old problems or misunderstandings, instantly finding one or more solutions through mediation or by highlighting communication problems between the partners that could condition the outcome of surgery and the resumption of intimacy for the two, avoiding sabotaging the medical and rehabilitation team, psychosexologist included.

Finally, the sexological anamnesis ascertains that there are no psychiatric or phobic pathologies, deviant behaviors, or self and heterodestructive practices.

9.4 Conclusions

Sexological anamnesis is also a form of self-learning for the patient. The psychosexologist's questions tend to make individuals reflect on their sexual, affective, and relational path and to understand their strengths and weaknesses.

Often, in fact, couples are not fully aware of their "culture of two" and take for granted every form of relationship and the presence of the other in their lives. The fear of surgery solicits the sense of belonging, the type of the emotional bond, the sense of protection and mutual care, the shared sense of responsibility in dealing with problematic situations, and not least their ability to "play".

This dimension is more nuanced in stable couples, and sexuality becomes a weekend appointment or an ultimatum after 3 weeks of abstinence.

Many of these couples reject routine sexuality made of ritualized gestures: to undress each other before bedtime, to shower together, to greet each other with an affectionate gesture (a caress), a passionate gesture (a kiss), and a mischievous gesture (a more impertinent touch) without "demanding a sexual performance at all costs."

Rediscovering the freedom to make the body a means of communication, without the obligation of sexual intercourse, frees partners from anxieties and fears and pushes them to experiment without criticism or judgment, a daily rediscovery of intimacy that can lead naturally to sexual intercourse without schedule or anxiety about fulfillment.

9.5 Sample Questionnaire for Andrological Anamnesis

These sample questions might be useful within the assessment of the medical history.

For the patient

- Did you ever experience bedwetting as a child or an adolescent?
- At what age did you experience the first spontaneous erection with ejaculation? (pollution)
- Do you remember whether it was day or night? What did you think then?
- At what age did you have your first complete sexual intercourse? Do you remember with whom? (friend, girlfriend of the moment, a foreign girl, etc.)
- Did you have any important relationships before your present one?
- How long did it last? Was it you who ended the relationship, or did they leave you? Do you remember the reasons it ended?
- Before meeting your current partner, how would you judge your sexuality?
- Have you ever suffered (even occasionally) from premature ejaculation, erectile dysfunction, drop in desire, or painful orgasm?
- How has your sexuality changed over time?
- Have you ever experienced fertility problems?

For the partner

- At what age did you have your first menstrual cycle (menarche)?
- Were you ready for this event?
- Every how many days does your monthly cycle fall?
- How many days does it last?
- Have you ever suffered from amenorrhea?
- Have you ever had gynecological surgery?
- When was your last menstrual cycle?
- At what age did you have your first complete sexual intercourse? Do you remember with whom?
- Did you have any important relationships before the present one?
- How long did it last? Was it you who ended the relationship, or did they leave you? Do you remember the reasons it ended?
- Before meeting your current partner, how would you judge your sexuality?
- Have you ever thought of trying to get pregnant?
- How would your partner react in such a situation?
- Who takes care of contraception?
- Have you ever had an abortion?
- How would you assess the quality of your sexuality today?

For the couple

- How does your partner seem? Worried, anxious?
- Did you find the prospect of surgery surprising?
- Which of you is most concerned about the surgical outcome?
- What do you expect from this intervention?
- How would you react (if you thought about it now) if the outcome of the intervention was not optimal?
- Which of you is familiar with the surgery?
- What do you expect from the surgical staff and during hospitalization?
- What do you fear most from doctors, nurses, and the psychosexologist?
- Who at this moment could well understand your feelings? (relatives, friends, acquaintances, no one, etc.)
- How do you see yourself in 5 years' time?
- How did you overcome small sexual failures during these years of cohabitation or marriage?
- Do you talk about your sexual desires?
- Which parts of your partner's body do you like best?

Reference

1. Derogatis LR, Kourlesis SM (1981) An approach to evaluation of sexual problems in the cancer patient. CA Cancer J Clin 31:46–50

Role of Informed Consent in Andrological Surgery in Adolescents and Adults

10

Mauro Silvani

10.1 Text

The legal medical aspect constitutes a topic of discussion among the heartiest members of the surgical medical profession, weighing heavily in andrological surgery, largely because of clinical diagnostic influences and therapeutic aspects which surgeons often balk at, in what is today called defensive medicine, with its useless investigations and admissions, and sensitivity to rising healthcare spending. In the last 10 years, the number of legal medical examiners has grown considerably, which has interfered with the doctor-patient relationship. Compensation claims for "malpractice" have increased from 200 to 500% in Italy, Spain, and Germany and 50% in the UK and the Scandinavian countries, but the concept of criminal liability in the health sector dates back to 1930 and that of civil liability to 1942. Informed consent is a fraudulent strategic path leading to surgery.

Consent to medical treatment makes legitimate any action of diagnosis, care, and assistance that otherwise would be unlawful (Cass. Pen. Sect. IV 14.3.2008 no. 11335). The first characteristic of a good informed consent form is the clarity and simplicity of exposition, which should contain a rich descriptive component, so as to make it understandable to anyone who wanted a consultation, and it should be delivered to the patient a few days before the intervention. Each consent form should then contain a part dedicated to the declaration of successful understanding of the pathology from which the patient is affected (Table 10.1) and one relating to the understanding and acceptance of the type of intervention suggested for the specific pathology (Table 10.2), which also illustrates the different available surgical solutions with the relative advantages and disadvantages of each possible option. This part of the consent form must describe the possible complications and how to resolve them. In the case of underage patients, signing the consent form must be done by either parent, and it is better if both set of parents do so, if they are separated, divorced, or a nonresident. The surgeon must always be the first operator to sign the consent form, although the presence of a witness from the medical team is not mandatory. The consent form thus collected is exhaustive both in

E. V. Longhi et al., *Psychosexual Counseling in Andrological Surgery*,
https://doi.org/10.1007/978-3-319-99646-2_10

Table 10.1 Expression of expected information

Facsimile
Date: …../…../……….
Signature and Doctor's stamp ____________________
Patient's signature (if an adult and able to understand and agree)____________________
Parent's or guardian's signature, confirming their identity (in the case of a minor patient)
____
Signature of the guardian, curator, or support administrator (whose identity has been verified and a copy of the protection provision, curation, or support administration acquired)
____
Possible patient signature (in case of curatorship or administration) ____________________

Table 10.2 Consent to the intervention by the patient

I, the undersigned, ____________________ born in ____________________, on ____________ declare that I have been informed in a clear and understandable way by Prof/Dr.________________________ that for the pathology diagnosed, the following intervention is indicated: …………………………………………………………………………………………
………
Having said this, I declare that I have been invited to read the above information form very carefully, which corresponds to what has been broadly and exhaustively explained to me orally. I also declare that I have understood the meaning of what has been shown to me and that I have no further clarifications to be advanced beyond those already provided to me. I am also aware that the type of surgery I consent to undergo may not be successful in treating the pathology in question.
However, I knowingly consent to the surgical treatment proposed to me and agree to respect all indications and recommended checks in the discharge letter.
Doctor's signature: ________________________________
Patient's signature: ________________________________
POSSIBLE NOTES…………………………………………………………………………………………

regard to understanding the pathology that is affecting the patient and for the proposed intervention for this pathology. Informed consent is, in any case, the last communicative step of a series of meetings between the patient, family, and medical team, which are aimed at developing an alliance and therapeutic concordance that is essential for deciding the best surgical option.

Communication with the patient must consider his comprehension skills to promote his participation and conscious adherence to the therapeutic diagnostic proposal. The information must be truthful yet limited to those elements that are acceptable to the patient's culture and psychological tradition, avoiding exaggeration of data and success rates [1]. This aspect is of special importance in cases of intervention for genital, testicular, or penile trauma in the case of priapism, in which the decision is communicated promptly to the patient and the family and in which the outcomes may sometimes not be favorable for fertility or erectile function [2–4].

The consensus will allow the patient to exercise his rights and make an effective assessment in this regard of the choices that are presented and illustrated. If the information is of such a nature as to cause suffering and anxiety, it must be provided with absolute clarity and circumspection with non-traumatic terminology and always with elements capable of leaving hope even if there is a poor chance of success. **Avoid passing from informed consent to terrorized consent.** Communication **must be personalized, tailored to the almost sartorial patient, especially for adolescents, a particularly vulnerable age group with which communication is sometimes difficult.** Information is the science of the doctor-patient relationship. The care relationship requires technical skills, but also dialogue, and the ability to incorporate protocols and schemes. The surgeon must also possess psychological skills that allow him to understand both the personality and the environmental situation of the patient to modulate the information provided [5]. Talks should not be fleeting, should number at least three before the intervention, and should have the purpose of explaining to the patient what surgery can and cannot do. In andrological surgery, patient expectations are very high in terms of aesthetic and functional results. The most fitting example in this regard is a request for penis enlargement in patients with long-established hard penises. These are patients with a retracted penis, a curved inelastic penis, one with an erectile deficiency, or a penis definable as having terminal organ disease, which require treatment beyond correction of the erectile dysfunction recurvatum and restoration of the native length of the shaft. In this case the surgeon will have to be very clear in communicating to the patient that the length of the shaft cannot be restored to its state before the disease even if this could lead the patient to choose another surgeon. In the case of an intervention for congenital recurvatum, the young patient will need to clearly understand that the shaft will undergo a shortening proportional to the degree of recurvatum. This type of problem will be illustrated and defined with particular clarity to an adolescent who often confronts and compares his genitals with models that generate false myths. Many other examples could be formulated. To better understand the characteristics of the ideal consensus, we report some of the detailed informed consensus and recommendations by the Italian Society of Andrology.

10.2 Conclusions

Informed consent in the surgical field is at the base of the doctor-patient relationship and, in addition to technical skills, is a further factor behind therapeutic success. It should not be interpreted as a means of protecting the doctor from possible judicial retaliatory action but rather as a tool for encouraging the patient's loyalty to the first clinical and therapeutic diagnostic path and then as a means to improve the patient's compliance, adherence, and therapeutic agreement. Correct information is the exact science of the pz (**Turillazzi**) medical report, and the full meaning of the communication is collected in a short and clear sentence. A well-executed operation may not be a success if the result is not what the patient expected; this can happen if the communication is hastily articulated in a single and fleeting comparison between the doctor and patient, perhaps the night before the surgery, with one-way communication in which the patient listens without the possibility of making a clarifying reply. Obtaining high-quality consent should be the goal of the surgeon before the procedure. He must possess simple and comprehensive speaking skills in illustrating the therapeutic pathway to the patient [6], yet above all, the consent required to administer it should be informed by national and/or international guidelines regarding the treatment of the pathology in question. Guidelines and informed consent represent two sides of the same coin in evidence-based medicine, whose principles must be inspired by medicine of the third millennium. To better understand the characteristics of the ideal consensus, we report some of the detailed informed consensus and recommendations by the Italian Society of Andrology.

References

1. Law of 28 March 2001 (ratification of the Oviedo Convention).
2. Lucky M, Brown G, Dorkin T, Pearcy R, Shabbir M, Shukla CJ, Rees RW, Summerton DJ, Muneer A, BAUS Section of Andrology and Genitourethral Surgery (AGUS) (2018) British Association of Urological Surgeons (BAUS) consensus document for the management of male genital emergencies—testicular trauma. BJU Int 121(6):840–844. https://doi.org/10.1111/bju.14163
3. Lucky M, Brown G, Dorkin T, Pearcy R, Shabbir M, Shukla CJ, Rees RW, Summerton DJ, Muneer A, BAUS Section of Andrology and Genitourethral Surgery (AGUS) (2018) British Association of Urological Surgeons (BAUS) consensus document for the management of male genital emergencies—penile fracture. BJU Int 122(1):26–28. https://doi.org/10.1111/bju.14167
4. Lucky M, Brown G, Dorkin T, Pearcy R, Shabbir M, Shukla CJ, Rees RW, Summerton DJ, Muneer A, BAUS Section of Andrology and Genitourethral Surgery (AGUS) (2018) BAUS consensus document for the management of male genital emergencies: priapism. BJU Int 121(6):835–839. https://doi.org/10.1111/bju.14140
5. National Bioethics Committee (1992)
6. Chiodi V et al (1973) Legal medicine manual. Vallardi ed, Milan

Part II

The Teenager and His Parents

11 Sexological Aspects Associated with Delayed Puberty and "Small Penis Syndrome"

The size of the penis, in many cultures, is synonymous with virility, power, dominance over men, and possession of women. A symbol of loving and being loved [1].

In some cases, such as in Egypt, sound sexual education has been helpful in dispelling myths and misconceptions about the size of the penis.

A study by Salama [2] of a sample of 239 young students (smokers and singles) reporting small penis, premature ejaculation, and even penile curvature showed that most of the penis sizes of patients were either normal or slightly below the lower indexes whether in flaccid or erect state. Generally though, not with truly small sexual organs.

There is more however. A study examined 20 patients with primary diagnosis of micropenis in childhood. Eight patients were diagnosed in prepuberty, between 10 and 13 years of age, and 12 patients between 17 and 43 years of age. All but one patient had been given gonadotropin, testosterone, or cortisone during childhood.

Only one child in the prepubertal group had a penis length above tenth percentile. All postpubertal patients had a member length below tenth percentile.

It transpired that puberty had been delayed in only two patients in the postpubertal group. All patients were heterosexual, and they achieved erection and orgasm. Eleven patients had ejaculations, 9 were sexually active, 7 were married, and 1 had fathered a child.

The research brings us so far. However, clinical experience in Italy shows that doubt about the size of the member is common among children, parents, and adults.

The first pediatric consultation, between 6 and 11 years of age, usually takes place in the presence of the mother, who is distressed by the difference in the size of the child's penis compared to his siblings, with a "hidden" sense of guilt that she did not bring up the child adequately compared to others. In the case of an only child, guilt for not being able to bear the perfect child.

E. V. Longhi et al., *Psychosexual Counseling in Andrological Surgery*,
https://doi.org/10.1007/978-3-319-99646-2_11

In a subsequent visit, the father also appears, expressing doubts about the future sexuality of the son. He feels somehow responsible, as a champion of the gender of the child, for possessing an abnormal virility, for being a bearer of inadequacy.

The frequent requests for clarification and reassurance from the parents to the doctor pertain to the normal growth and sexuality of the child, but it is also often a disguised request for "absolution" on the part of the father and mother as "normal parents."

The teenager, independently, is assailed by doubt arising from comparisons with peers, especially when in the changing rooms, "collective dramas" are fed (my basketball teammates in the changing rooms called me "nib" because they said that I had a small penis ...); triggering in the youth and his family calls for clinical consultations and quick medical solutions.

Let us not forget obese children. The Istituto Superiore di Sanità (Higher Institute of Health) recently announced that one child (6–11 years old) in three in Italy is above average weight: 22% overweight and 13% obese. About 25% of overweight young people have an obese parent, and 34% have both overweight parents.

Here, consultation at the psychological level appears more complex. The child's small penis is nothing more than an "anomaly" for the parent with respect to the child's body shape. Round, ponderous, strong, and with a disproportionate, inadequate, nonexistent virility. Sometimes hidden in the folds of fat on the abdomen.

The so-called buried penis, as defined by Maizels, is hidden under the preputial skin. This may be caused by excessive fat in the prepubic area of the anterior abdominal wall or by the lack of anchoring of the surface fascia and skin to the deepest fascia at the base of the penis.

The term "buried penis" was first used by Keyes in 1919. Crawford has differentiated a buried penis secondary to an excess of suprapubic fat that could improve with age from a penis that is buried following superficial fascial laxity, which commonly requires surgical correction.

Abnormal bands have also been described between the fascia of Scarpa and the Buck's fascia that binds the penis. Large scrotal masses such as hernias and/or hydrocells may also bury the penis.

Excessive preputial skin (megaprepuce) is another circumstance where the penis appears to be buried (under a large amount of foreskin). It is important to remember that the penis shaft in these children is normal, and excessive redundancy or abnormal anchoring of the surrounding tissue would result in a relatively decreased penis size.

That said, to avoid confusion, there are two main classifications of reference: Crawford (with three main forms of small penis) and Maizels (who describes four):

11.1 Crawford

1. Concealed penis
2. Buried penis
3. Webbed penis
4. Photo (**a**–**c**)

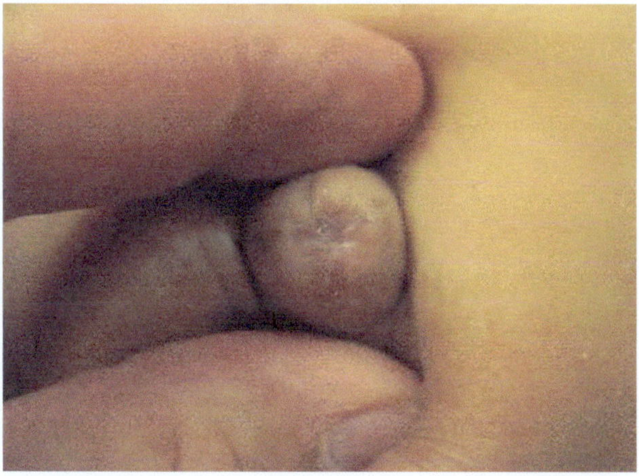

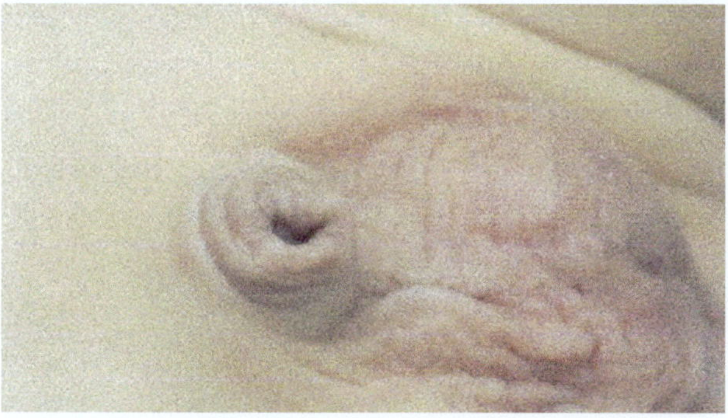

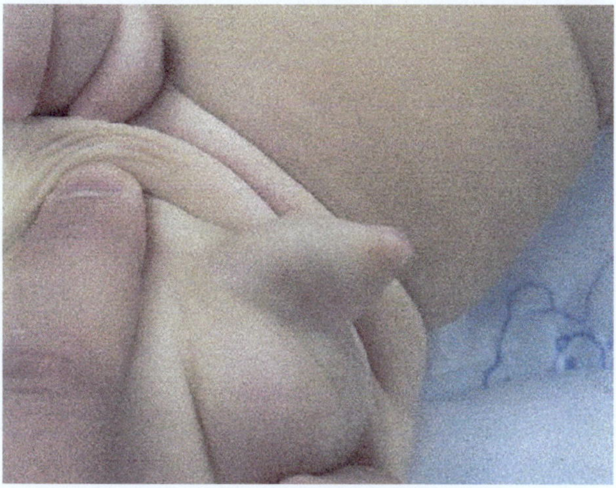

11.2 Maizels

1. *Buried*: in the newborn the penis shaft is buried, as it is in early childhood, by the skin of the pubis, while in the teenager, it is buried in the prepubic fat.
2. *Webbed*: the skin of the scrotum and penis are not separated.
3. *Trapped*: the penis is trapped due to trauma or to the effects of circumcision.
4. *Micropenis: the only form in which there is a real small size of the length and girth of the penis*
   According to David Veale, psychiatrist and head of the research team at King's College London, the small penis is an idea that "is all in the head".

Like other forms of dissatisfaction with body shape (weight, height, muscles), anxiety about a small penis rarely has any real clinical confirmation. As irrational as it is, insecurity surrounding the small penis sometimes hides "repressed trauma" because (as Veale maintains) "some boys were ridiculed unfairly by a former partner or by a teenager in the showers in the gym or in the changing room."

In contrast, a survey published in the journal *Proceedings of National Academy of Sciences* (April, 2011) questioned the myth of the super gifted, revealing that women would not be particularly impressed when faced with a (flaccid) penis longer than 8.5 cm.

A study published in the Journal of Sexual Medicine in 2012 also found that the size of the member made a difference only to women with habitual vaginal orgasms. For other partners, size does not matter.

11.3 Micropenis

Micropenis is defined as a member of normal morphology, whose length is 2.5 standard deviations from the mean, by age and by stage of sexual development, in the absence of associated pathologies or abnormalities.

The first description of normal penis length, in relation to the age of development (from birth to adulthood), dates back to a 1942 publication by Schonfeld and Beebe.

Micropenis is found in males with genital organs compatible with karyotype 46 XY and may be associated with scrotum hypoplasia and non-descent of the testicles. The hypoplasia of the corpora cavernosa and the spongy body changes its aesthetic appearance, also causing a significant reduction in diameter.

In most cases, micropenis is caused by reduced testosterone secretion, which occurs in the second and third trimesters of uterine life, for reasons mostly unknown. When reduced testosterone secretion occurs as early as the first trimester, hypospadias and more severe sexual development defects (sexual differentiation disorders, DSD) are associated with micropenis.

Micropenis is also observed in many malformation syndromes and in the congenital deficit of growth hormone (GH). Episodes of hypoglycemia at birth and poor growth from the first months of life are manifestations of congenital deficiency or insensitivity to GH.

On a psychological level, many parents of GH-deficient infants are followed by andrologists and endocrinologists, but it is not yet a routine practice to make a psychological referral.

The parents often see the child as deformed, handicapped, and lacking a quality of life identical to other infants. Parents experience anxiety and resentment toward an undeserved and discriminatory existential injustice.

Most of them appear to be zealous and overprotective, but communication with the doctor often alternates between modes of subjection and communication styles that could lead to the presumption of distrust toward specialists and anger toward their own impotence.

No clinic, or almost no clinic, other than by its own inclination, is culturally prepared to read these ambivalent manifestations. Most of the time, parents ask how to "read the cries or the caprices" of their newborn babies. They are told that "newborns don't have caprices, they only have needs."

11.3.1 Which?

Often these children appear shy and emotionally retarded and exhibit behaviors undermining of authority. Only in the school and prepubertal age do parents have clear evidence of the discomfort of the child and the delay in growth, including in emotionality, character, emotional relationships, development of identity, and the sexual role.

Micropenis becomes of secondary importance, as parents feel that their child is growing through constant care and sexually evolving through clinical examinations and pharmacotherapy. *The unease of the child and the parent, however, often goes unheard.*

In the future, research protocols and integrated approaches between andrologist, endocrinologist, and psychosexologist should be set up to allow clinicians and any family with a GH-deficit child to bring up the child with individualized projects.

11.4 Conclusion

Normal values of penile length from birth to adulthood (Feldman and Smith, 1975-Flatau, 1975-Schonfeld and Beebe, 1942)

Age	Mean ± SD	Mean ± 2.5 SD
Infant 30 weeks	2.5 ± 0.4	1.5
Infant 34 weeks	3.0 ± 0.4	2.0
0–5 months	3.9 ± 0.8	1.9
6–12 months	4.3 ± 0.8	2.3
1–2 years	4.7 ± 0.8	2.6
2–3 years	5.1 ± 0.9	2.9
3–4 years	5.5 ± 0.9	3.3
4–5 years	5.7 ± 0.9	3.5

Age	Mean ± SD	Mean ± 2.5 SD
5–6 years	6.0 ± 0.9	3.8
6–7 years	6.1 ± 0.9	3.9
7–8 years	6.2 ± 1.0	3.7
8–9 years	6.3 ± 1.0	3.8
9–10 years	6.3 ± 1.0	3.8
10–11 years	6.4 ± 1.1	3.7
Adult	13.3 ± 1.6	9.3

The literature and clinical research show that the average size of the male penis is 9.16 cm in length, and 9.13 cm in circumference when the organ is flaccid, and 13.12 cm in length, by 11.66 cm in circumference when erect. Exceptions to the average are quite rare: only 5 men out of 100 have genitalia longer than 16 cm, and only 5 out of 100 have a penis shorter than 10 cm. The length considered is from the pubic bone to the tip of the glans, excluding skin folds or centimeters of fat.

Although the tables and clinical studies are constantly evolving, small penis syndrome refers not only to body dysmorphism but also to identity problems that often result (in puberty) in food, alcohol, and drug dependency.

At best, reasoning with a boy with this syndrome allows you to quell anxieties and fears, not to mention undisclosed creeping depressions.

Although the topic may make non-clinicians smile, the suffering of these young patients is very deep. Talking with one's parents about small penis syndrome is difficult; with one's peers it is impossible.

Doctors, as much as they may embarrass a young patient, are the "most neutral" and uncritical interlocutors.

Excessive normalization "don't worry, everything is fine" is often not enough to alleviate an anxiety that goes beyond the aesthetic and sexual aspect.

A supposedly small penis leads to the doubt "will I be a powerful man? To what extent can I consider myself fit to face the world?"

Every boy is waiting to be able to answer these questions with the support of clinicians and psychosexologists: not without being able to talk about their anxieties and emotional upsets.

Case Illustration

Johann is a 16-year-old boy, the youngest of three. The shyest, the most graceful, and the most awkward with girls. He asked for an andrological visit because he reported having suffered from night enuresis between the ages of 5 and 8, until the pediatrician advised his parents, because of his reserved and introverted nature, to join a rugby team. Today he is afraid he has a small and "sick" penis. At the andrological examination, the doctor diagnosed genital psoriasis and a member in the group norm. He prescribed dermatological and psychosexological examinations and advice.

"My first erection with ejaculation," he begins, "was just after a great try in the third match of the Junior League. I was 13...my teammates took the mickey on the pitch. They called me 'drop' ... and in the dressing rooms, they threw me fully dressed into the shower" "Drop is the nickname that I still carry, even though I now play in Serie B."

Sport was a "great outlet" for Johann "I was finally someone. My brothers had always been champions of everything: top of the class, ski champions, climbing, swimming. Because of my kyphosis, up to the age of 8 I was doing corrective gymnastics three times a week ... Then my triumph. The junior rugby league. I was finally someone. Even if at home they called me 'small'... until that tragic summer...."

Johann says that one summer, he was a guest of a teammate in Forte dei Marmi, Tuscany, and he finally felt he had a physique to behold. But one afternoon "while I was in the bath, my team-mate's sister enters the bathroom, Ginevra 19 years old, and cries out "Mamma mia, what a small one..." Johann feels embarrassed, stutters something, and then shouts at her to leave the room. He is worried, embarrassed, and, the same evening, makes an excuse to call home to be picked up.

Why do you remember all this? He hasn't had full sexual intercourse yet, because he fears losing the girl. "Miriam cheers for me and my team: she's the most desired girl but if she then "sees how small it is"...she could tell everyone...I always put on my costume when I take a shower in the changing rooms and my teammates call me "lifeguard"...but if they were to see my penis...I'd be finished."

It is clear that Johann's psoriasis at the genital level is a way to "protect" the small penis and to ward off all possibilities of confrontation. Johann still seems to suffer the comparison with his brothers. They are now at University; Johann preferred the hotel school. He wants to travel the world, become a great chef, not get married, stay single, and be a winner on his own.

In fact, the size of the penis is normal, but the reassurances of the andrologist sound like "an alliance between men. A way to reassure me ... but the girls criticize you ..." He confesses to have tried a commercial relationship, but in the end, I just talked because I was embarrassed. Matilde, the escort, told me I'm normal...but they say that to all the customers, don't they?

When I ask Johann, "How many tries will you have to score on the field to humiliate all your opponents and punish them because they would be better sexually with Miriam?" Johann reddens and explains that he is tired of escaping from sexuality and girls. Punishment is effected by avoiding autoeroticism, by rubbing the member only with the pillow or the sheet. "I'm dirty, and I feel depressed until I get onto the pitch. A few minutes of ecstasy on the pitch and then I fall back into the fear of being discovered and that everyone knows that I have a small penis."

Psoriasis, small penis, depression, inadequacy, and fear of being happy. These are the themes proposed to Johann on which to work with the psychosexologist: I, a woman, for the first time, who is uncritical and who with him would have built a therapeutic path, without losers or winners. Without rivalry, with only the objective of a second "human project." With a goodbye to "drop, small, lifeguard."

11.5 Medical History Questions

- How long have you had this idea?
- Do you remember an event, a fact, and a criticism that may have influenced your doubt?
- Do you have a girlfriend?
- At what age did you have your first pollution? What did you think at the time? Were you prepared, or did you only have information "by hearsay" from your friends?
- Who knows of your doubt?
- How much time do you spend each day on this thought?
- If you woke up tomorrow morning with a more satisfying penis, how would your life change?
- How much do you masturbate? Do you feel pleasure, or do other not always pleasant sensations get in the way?
- What are you afraid could happen in the future because of the "small penis?"
- What unexpected positive things could happen?
- What expectations did you have about this consultation?

11.6 Self-Check

There are no right or wrong answers. This is just a way to see ourselves outside of the clinical context.

When you meet a young patient who complains of small penis syndrome, do you tend to:

1. Sympathize with the boy.
2. Reassure the parent, if he/she accompanies him.
3. Underestimate the fear and anxiety of the patient.
4. Hide your irritation in the face of a trivial problem.
5. Worry about not being able to be useful except with the andrological visit.
6. Send him as soon as possible to the psychosexologist.
7. Talk to the boy about his sexuality.
8. Identify the trauma that may have caused the syndrome.
9. Dismiss him as soon as possible and conclude the visit with a "mollifying" letter.
10. Ask him come back after a month to verify his state of mind.

References

1. Talalaj J et al (1994) The strangest human sex, ceremonies and customs. Hill of Content, Melbourne
2. Salama N (2016) Consultations for small penis in Egyptian males. Am J Mens Health 10(3):220–227

Surgical Correction of Symptomatic Varicocele in Adolescents

12

Elena Vittoria Longhi and Fabio Ferro

Varicocele is the expansion of the veins of the pampiniform plexus that drains the testicle. Varicocele is found in 15% of men. Of these, 19–41% will have primary infertility, and 45–81% will have secondary infertility.

In couple's infertility the problem is attributable to male in 20% of cases and in 27% to both. It is not possible to identify the cause in 15% of male and female. When the male is finally considered the cause of infertility, in 1–2% the problem is secondary to hypogonadism, in 10–20% to post-testicular defects (disorders of sperm transport), 40–50% due to nonclassifiable disorders, and in 30–40% ascribable to testicular diseases (primary spermatogenesis failure and hypogonadism). Between congenital disorders: Klinefelter syndrome, cryptorchidism, miotonic dystrophy, congenital anorchia (vanishing testis), androgenic insensitivity S., 5-alpha-reductase deficiency, and Y chromosome deletions and varicocele (V). The prevalence of V is 15% of male population. The dilation of scrotal veins became evident during adolescence for the evident dimorphism, but the predisposition is congenital with a genetic component. Familiarity (first-degree relative affected by varicocele) increases the prevalence up to 50%. The varicocele's influence on fertility derives from its presence in about 40% of males with primary infertility and in 80% with secondary infertility. The V is considered the most common correctable etiology found in adults with infertility (Goldstein J Urol 1995), but there is still a great debate about its treatment and the positive impact on fertility. Few reports outline how varicocele has an impact not only on fertility, which is already an important cause of anxiety and depression itself, but especially in those characterized by a history of many unsuccessful attempts with reproductive technology. In fact, possible psychological consequences can derive from the evident scrotal dysmorphism, especially in adolescents, for decline of testosterone, precocious andropause, and the couple disharmony. The fig … shows the events who can determine male depression.

Most varicocele in adolescents are diagnosed during a routine medical examination, and it is difficult to predict which of these children will show a decreased testicular function in adulthood. As in adults, surgical treatment of varicocele is the

E. V. Longhi et al., *Psychosexual Counseling in Andrological Surgery*,
https://doi.org/10.1007/978-3-319-99646-2_12

most recognized treatment. However, unlike an adult varicocelectomy, treatment for an adolescent varicocele is more often laparoscopic. The treatment objectives are the same for both adolescent and adult patients.

In the treatment of adolescent varicocele, the surgeon generally tries to prevent testicular injury and maintain the function of the testicle to protect future fertility.

In a small percentage of adolescents, varicocele has a detrimental effect on testicular growth and can lead to irreversible testicular damage.

There is no consensus in the literature on the time limit of commencement of treatment in adolescents with varicocele, nor on what method to use. It therefore seems that the most important problem for andrologist surgeons in the management of adolescent varicocele is to select patients who actually need treatment.

That said the impact of this surgery on the young person is more easily described years later, for example, during a psychosexological visit, as in the case of Francesco.

12.1 Clinical Case

Francesco, 24, has had a partner Enrica, 21, for a short time. “I decided late to have a partner because sex seemed to me a painful and complicated experience,” he said to andrologist. “It disgusts me to take my penis in my hand; during the relationship I can’t penetrate Enrica ....I had to talk about it with someone, because I felt so bad ....”

The fear of losing the bond with his partner brought Francesco to finally face the problem (as the young man describes his decision). During the sexual anamnesis following the andrological examination, I ask the patient if this hostile feeling toward his member is dictated by a particular event or moment. And the story becomes “a river in full flow”:

“At the age of 13, my uncle, a doctor, consulted by my mother, convinced my parents to get to the bottom of my problem. I didn’t understand anything about medical terms, my uncle spoke about varicocele, and I immediately thought it was a terrible disease. My mother continued to say that in her family, there had never been ‘a man other than a man,’ and she continued to cry. My father pretended it was nothing, “stay calm, he told me, you’re in good hands. Your uncle (the brother of his father) is a doctor and knows what to do..... In practice my uncle did everything. He took me to a colleague for a medical visit. They talked to each other, as if I weren’t there...Every now and then my uncle looked at me and smiled at me...I thought they were hiding something from me...Strangely, the other doctor when greeting me said ‘everything’s fine’, your uncle will take care of you.”

“At that moment,” continues Francesco, “my uncle didn’t say anything about the visit except ‘You see? Nothing happened!’, but once we had returned home, he locked himself in my father’s study and spoke at length with my parents. My father, an architect, spoke little and in a low voice. I only heard my mother crying... A week later I was in the hospital, and they operated on me. I saw that event as a violation, a castration, a family conspiracy...Not to mention the dressings that my uncle gave me at home, then staying for dinner or lunch with us, as if nothing had happened.

I hated them for a long time, I closed in on myself. I didn't look at my genitals, I would take a shower and try to think that when I was 18 years and 1-day old, I would leave home...."

Francesco has never had a full sexual relationship, he has always maintained affective relationships with girls, but without sex, "and for this reason, I lost all of them" he explained. Until Enrica, his university friend at the Faculty of Architecture, arrived "and now I feel in love, and I don't want to lose her, like my mother did."

Francesco's mother, who had become pregnant, was left by her then fiancé 1 week before the wedding. "She always feels guilty for everything," the patient points out, and "we lived for 5 years with my maternal grandparents." Then Giovanni, my father, arrived, almost by chance. A colleague of my mother, a young graduate architect, recently hired in the same design studio. I don't remember anything, my mother told me about it. I only remember that Giovanni corrected my maths homework...When I was 9, we went to live with Giovanni and all his family. Engineers, surveyors, architects...our life suddenly became more cheerful and with more people visiting...My mother suddenly became more beautiful, more groomed... and I thought "she's never done that for me"...then along came Giovanni's doctor brother, the family "guru." He spoke and everyone obeyed. I became fond of him and thought, "If I am loved by my powerful uncle, I will become powerful! At home, until he betrayed me... He made me have the operation without consulting me, without explaining anything to me, except "You are lucky Francesco, you can have a wife and children like all men," "What do I want with a wife and children at 13 years old, I thought and here I am, afraid of losing Enrica."

Francesco, in the course of his anamnesis, reveals that he has difficulty in exciting himself and feeling pleasure. Enrica is with him. She listens to the whole story, and in the end, I ask "did you know about all this?" "Not everything," answers the partner, "but I'm glad he opened up. I too am a virgin, and Francesco doesn't have faith in his potential..."

What can be drawn from this? Certainly, Francesco has suffered a physical, psychic, and relational trauma. He feels the burden of "being a man at all costs" in that family, to absolve an abandoned mother who "did not know how to keep a man close." And not least, "so as not to disappoint the expectations of a father, Giovanni, who gave him his name and who has always raised him as a natural son." It is a pity that to Francesco's questions about who his natural father was, his mother always answered "you haven't missed anything, he has already made me suffer."

The trauma of surgery emphasized an already quite weak idea of virile power, and the uncle's arrogance (as Francesco calls it) was experienced as much more than a deception: an abuse, a violation, a condemnation of non-virility for life. Or at least this is how Francesco saw it.

Today he doesn't want to repeat his mother's family script, and thanks to Enrica, he is trying to fill an affective void, a missed masculine role, a possibility for two to live with projects and desires "long term" (as Enrica describes it).

12.1.1 The Rationale of the Parents and of the Doctor

Although he has only the memory of Francesco and his later descriptions, it is clear that Giovanni's family system has tried to compensate in every way for the failure of the patient's mother. It was certainly the first secure family nucleus (after that of the maternal grandparents), with a strong sense of belonging, where problems are solved in-house.

All these graduates and successful professionals provided Francesco and his mother with a new social status, a new successful future. His doctor uncle seems to be the reference person for everyone as well as being the one who takes responsibility for uncomfortable and unpopular roles inside and outside the house. To defend the fragility of Francesco's mother and of the whole family.

Perhaps the mother could have nourished a sense of inadequacy in the face of such family efficiency, but it is certain that Francesco's diagnosis of varicocele may have awakened old wounds of pain and despondency, in a woman "adopted" in full by Giovanni and his family. Giovanni, his father, is described as a serene, sweet, affectionate man by Francesco, someone who went with him to play soccer and followed him in all the soccer tournaments.

His uncle was perhaps the most authoritative voice only because he was the only doctor in the midst of engineers and architects. Also because he was trusted by all the family members in cases of "illnesses, pains, or simple fears" as Francesco ironically describes.

Importantly, however, the doctor uncle had lost a child, a cot death: his only child. What projections could this uncle have on Francesco? Is it possible that he felt he could redeem the child he had never seen grow up? And a father's role so little lived? Francesco had not realized then, as he does not now that he had more than one father, too intent on redeeming everything and everyone through him. Perhaps it was too much for a young teenager, whose "guilt" was to have been conceived too early. And he hadn't had the time to choose a manly role just for himself.

12.1.2 The Andrologist Surgeon's Rationale

We do not have Francesco's medical record, and we cannot reconstruct the diagnostic process and the reasons for surgical treatment. However, as we know, doctors often talk to doctors and take it for granted that the colleague who goes home then reports information, news, with equal professionality to family members.

Or perhaps his medical uncle, solid in his role, in an attempt to protect everyone, unconsciously excluded Francesco and his sensitivity as a young man in the making.

Take-Home Messages

What we can draw from everyone's reasoning is that an intervention for varicocele in a teenager involves the whole family history. The impact of surgery on the young patient cannot be separated from the affective, emotional, and relational ties with parents and the most authoritative members of the family.

Each of them brings the surgeon an emotional diagnosis which, if it remains undetected, risks creating conflict, anguish, and symmetry in the family relationship and in the intimacy of the adolescent.

It is important that every surgeon should have interviews with adolescents and parents before treatment: to share the clinical-surgical approach with the help of drawings. To frame, with the help of the psychosexologist, the implications of such surgery in the intimacy of the young patient and family.

Medical advice alone cannot create a lasting safe outcome for a teenager and for the adult of tomorrow. This at least seems to be what Francesco's doctor uncle teaches us.

12.2 Conclusion

The treatment of varicocele in an adolescent presents many complexities to be assessed individually on a case-by-case basis. In addition to diagnosis and clinical treatment, the surgeon's emotion is also evident when faced with different types of adolescent characters and different types of parents.

The moment of birth, as does a surgical event for a child, disrupts the whole family system. Ignoring states of mind, family roles, and unconscious projections of the parents' history on the child, as in the case of Francesco, cancels out the purpose of the treatment and the purpose of the same.

Surgeon, teenager, family and psychosexologist can over time, form a team of therapists, some aware, others less aware (teenagers and parents), who participate in the making of a health experience, an opportunity for sharing and positive planning.

12.3 Self-Check

There are no answers which are more correct than others. There are ways, styles, and sensations that every surgeon needs to know in order to turn his or her knowledge into an effective therapeutic process:

1. When you see a teenager, are the parents present?
2. How would you change the way you evaluate the goal of your visit if you were alone with the teenager?

3. When you reveal the diagnosis, to whom does your gaze most frequently turn?
4. Are you more concerned about being scientifically correct or about providing information in a simple way?
5. If you draw the eventual pathology or surgical treatment, to whom do you give the drawing at the end of the visit?
6. If a teenager shows you hostility, what is your first reaction?
7. At what point in the diagnostic process would you consult the psychosexologist?
8. If one of the parents seems to underestimate the situation, what is your first reaction?

12.4 Medical History Questions

12.4.1 For the Adolescent

1. You seemed most attentive during the explanation: What was the sensation you felt most?
2. If you could choose a solution for varicocele, what would you recommend to the andrologist?
3. Which of your parents seems more worried?
4. What do you think could happen, both positive and less positive things, after the treatment that the andrologist explained?
5. If your brothers (sisters) were here, what would they think about the situation?
6. Who would you tell if you were afraid or worried about the outcome of the treatment?
7. Who would you like with you right now?

12.4.2 For the Parents

1. How do you see the situation?
2. What do you think about the treatment proposed by the andrologist?
3. How do you think your son will react?
4. What do you fear most about your son's reaction?
5. With whom does he speak more (the father or the mother)?
6. (In case of siblings) How do you plan to inform the other children? Will you do this in the presence of your son or separately?
7. Who will inform your family about the treatment planned for the varicocele of your child?
8. How will you justify the absence of your child, at school, at swimming....?
9. What thoughts most often pass through your mind in this period?
10. What worries you about your son's future?

Bibliography

1. Diamond DA et al (2011) Current management principles for adolescent varicocele. Fertil Steril 96:1294–1298
2. Dohle GR et al (2013) How common are varicoceles? New data on the prevalence in adolescence and new discussions. Andrology 1:661–662
3. Garolla A et al (2015) Twenty-four-hour monitoring of scrotal temperature in obese men and men with a varicocele as a mirror of spermatogenic function. Hum Reprod 30:1006–1013
4. Kass EJ et al (2001) Varicocele in adolescence induces left and right testicular volume loss. BJU Int 87:499–501
5. Kass EJ et al (2003) The adolescent varicocele: treatment and outcome. Curr Urol Rep 3:100–106
6. Chiba K et al (2016) Varicocele: diagnostic dilemmas, challenges and future prospects. Asian J Androl 18(2):276–281
7. Kumanov P et al (2008) Adolescent varicocele: who is at risk? Pediatrics 121:53–57
8. Kurtz MP et al (2015) Semen parameters in adolescents with varicocele: association with testis volume differential and total testis volume. J Urol 193:1843–1847
9. Lee YJ et al (2015) Usefulness of 2010 World Health Organization reference values for determining indications for varicocelectomy. Urology 85:831–835
10. Li F et al (2012) Effect of varicocelectomy on testicular volume in children and adolescents: a meta-analysis. Urology 79:1340–1345
11. Oster J et al (1971) Varicocele in children and adolescents. An investigation of the incidence among Danish school children. Scand J Urol Nephrol 5:27–32
12. Patuszack AW et al (2014) Diagnostic and management approaches to pediatric and adolescent varicocele: a survey of pediatric urologists. Urology 84:450–455
13. Robinson SP et al (2010) Treatment strategy for the adolescent varicocele. Urol Clin North Am 37:269–278
14. Skoog SJ et al (1997) The adolescent varicocele: what's new with an old problem in young patients? Pediatrics 100:112–121
15. Van Batavia JP et al (2010) Adolescent varicocele: influence of Tanner stage at presentation on the presence, development, worsening and/or improvement of testicular hypotrophy without surgical intervention. J Urol 184:731–734
16. Zampieri N et al (2007) Varicocele and adolescents: semen quality after 2 different laparoscopic procedures. J Androl 28:727–733
17. Silber SJ (2001) The varicocele dilemma. Hum Reprod Update 1:70–77
18. Tulloch JW (1952) A consideration of sterility factors in the light of subsequent pregnancies: subfertility in the male. Trans Edinb Obstet 59:29
19. Jungwirth A et al (2012) Guidelines for the investigation and treatment of male infertility. European Association of Urology

13 Monorchidism, Anorchidism, and Testicular Prosthesis in Children and Adolescents

Elena Vittoria Longhi and Alessandro Franceschelli

Unilateral anorchidism or monorchidism refers to the absence of a testicle. It is defined as the partial or complete absence, unilateral or bilateral, of the testicular tissue, with or without remains of the epididymis and the sperm cord, in the presence of internal development of the Wolffian duct and normal genitalia.

It is believed that ischemia due to intrauterine testicular torsion is the cause of monorchidism and therefore is a syndrome of testicular regression.

Children's sexual identity can be distorted by anomalies involving the genital area. The awareness of being male is normally considered as established after the third year of life. For these reasons, the most appropriate age to perform a prosthesis insertion should be as low as possible. This leads to peculiar technical problems: before puberty the scrotum is not developed yet, sometimes even hypoplastic because of the gonad absence, with prosthesis and scrotum disproportion. Implanting a small device reduces the risk of extrusion, but the prosthesis needs to be changed following child's growth. Risks resulting from an overdistended sac are ischemia of the scrotal wall and extrusion, although this complication seems to be more related to technical misleads than to the noncompliant scrotal sac. Indications for testicular prosthesis are not uncommon in children and adolescents: cryptorchidism (vanishing testis, testis to be removed because too high for an orchidopexy, postoperative atrophy), acute scrotum (spermatic cord torsion, strangulated groin hernia, trauma, orchitis), dysgenetic gonads, and tumors are all causes for an absent testis [1]. Recent studies demonstrated that TP are well accepted in adult patients (Turek, Ashead, Bodiwala, Henderson), and no induced systemic diseases were referred [2–4]. The majority of patients who had a prosthesis implanted reported an improvement in body image, and preserved self-esteem, sexual life, and performance were not compromised by TP (Table 13.1).

Different techniques for testicular prosthesis insertion are described; all of them are thought to facilitate the implant, to minimize complication, and to achieve good cosmetic results. In spite of young age and growth deals. Pediatric patients should be considered as a challenge to insert a prosthesis which won't need to be changed.

E. V. Longhi et al., *Psychosexual Counseling in Andrological Surgery*,
https://doi.org/10.1007/978-3-319-99646-2_13

Table 13.1

Diagnosis	*n* (%)
Vanished testis	193 (51.9%)
Atrophy post-orchidopexy	66 (17.7%)
Spermatic cord torsion	68 (18.3%)
Strangulated groin hernia	10 (2.7%)
Tumor-leukemia	19 (5.1%)
Atrophy post-herniotomy	15 (5%)
Hypogonadism (Kallmann S., Klinfelter S.)	3 (0.8%)
DSD	6 (1.6%)
Atrophy post cecal appendectomy	2 (0.5%)
Trauma	1 (0.27%)
Substitution for displacement (implanted elsewhere)	1 (0.27%)
Total	TP in 372 patients

We used three different techniques for TP insertion, depending on the age, the scrotal volume, the cause of mono-anorchidism, and an eventual previous surgery.

Approach 1: Related to the main cause of monorchidism and anorchidism (vanishing testis), our policy is to insert an artificial testis of medium size (20–21 mL) at the moment of primary school. Due to disproportion between scrotum and prosthesis, the approach is via an inguinal incision to avoid any scrotal wall wound [5]. In the majority of cryptorchid patients, a pre-existing inguinal scar is present because of previous surgery. Once the superficial inguinal fascia is opened, through this incision a digital scrotal distension is performed. TP, accurately rinsed in saline solution without antibiotics, is inserted and pushed into the sac through the surgical plane created between the superficial inguinal fascia and the muscle plane. A secondary skin incision is made at the scrotal root; a small extra dartoic fascia pouch is created, and one suture (polyglactin 0 or 2/0) is applied dartos to dartos in order to close the entrance of the scrotal neck. This approach allows avoiding the obstacle of pubis bone which makes it impossible or very difficult applying the stich from the inguinal wound side.

Approach 2: In postpubertal patients, when the scrotum is adequate to allocate a large prosthesis, we use a small modification of the technique described by Libman [6]. The incision is performed directly on the scrotal root instead of laterally to the penis, as originally described. The sutures to close the scrotal entrance are easy to apply, and the scar is not visible. The general anesthesia is combined to a local block. Local anesthesia is the standard protocol in collaborating with patients. The dartoic fascia is opened and, if required, the spermatic cord and testicular remnant excised. After TP is introduced, the scrotal entrance is closed approximating the dartos with 3/0 or 4/0 polyglactin suture.

Approach 3: As previously described, in patients with hypogonadism with two hypotrophic testes, an alternative technique is used. The surgical approach is done along the scrotal raphe. The two vaginal sacs are carefully dissected from the dartos preserving intact the scrotal septum. The spermatic cord of one side is released up to external inguinal ring, and the testes are moved to the opposite hemiscrotum through a small window of the high scrotal septum and sutured on the opposite gonad with fine sutures approximating the opened tunicas vaginalis. The testes are pexied to the dartos, and the TP is then inserted in the opposite hemiscrotum. The scrotal septum is sutured together with the dartos of the scrotal wall [7].

Elder reports only one complication out of 41 cases: a superficial infection that did not necessitate removal of the prosthesis, but his series counted only six pediatric patients [8].

13.1 How and When to Intervene

The questions of "how and when" to intervene, however, are still open.

Peycelon M. [9] in the article "Testicular prosthesis in children: Is earlier better?" published in the Journal of Pediatric Urology points out that the lack of a testicle in children occurs often and for various reasons but that the implantation of testicular prosthesis in these cases is very rare.

The most difficult decision is often made by parents, who rely on their instinct to evaluate whether a testicular prosthesis should be implanted into a preschool or adolescent child.

Unless they are confronted with an acute episode, such as the twisting of the only testicle, this will lead them to take urgent action and then, reluctantly, to plan other operations and further anesthesia to adapt the prosthesis when the son reaches adolescence.

Not all males with a single testicle need to have a testicular prosthesis implant.

For the clinicians, the absence of a testicle per se does not signal the necessity of prosthetic implantation, as many males do not seem disturbed by the lack of a testicle and may still feel satisfied with their body image.

Daily clinical experience shows that there is a great divergence of feeling between adolescent and adult males about the desire and need for testicular prosthetic implant.

Luca Incroci's 1999 retrospective study of the body image and sexual functioning of these patients showed that of 30 patients between the ages of 18 and 47 (with a silicone gel testicular prosthesis (TP)), 80% reported no sexual problems, 20% felt uncomfortable with intimate intercourse, 68% found an improvement in body image, and 45% reported premature ejaculation.

The hospital clinic shows that during periods when testicular prostheses were not on the market, some adolescents exhibited mood disorders, self-destructiveness, severe depression, and even suicidal behavior.

Moreover, those patients with monorchidism observe over time an increasingly reduced and asymmetric scrotum, which, if not a direct source of body dysmorphism, becomes an implicit cause of shame, discomfort, and a feeling of otherness in everyday life.

And not only in hygiene practices and intimacy.

On the other hand, with regard to child testicular prosthesis, Elder JS [10] published a study on 41 children under the age of 5. Testicular prostheses were implanted, with these results:

1. One complication for superficial wound infection without removal of the prosthesis.
2. Two boys reported slight scrotal discomfort.
3. In the long-term follow-up, 91% of families considered the aesthetic aspect to be good.
4. Ninety-four percent were satisfied with the decision to implant a prosthesis.

Certainly only an even longer-term follow-up could allow us to understand:

1. What memories of the prosthetic intervention these former children have, once they are adolescents and/or adults?
2. What sensations were left in the emotional memory of the young adults?
3. Sensations during sexual intercourse.
4. Reactions from partners.
5. The degree of gratification of one's own body image.

However, even Weissbach L [11] agrees that the crucial factor of the recommendation for the implantation of a prosthetic testicle is "the psychological and mental state of the patient." His study publishes the results of a questionnaire on 88 patients with testicular prosthesis, in which it emerges that males, before surgery, suffered "from a form of incompleteness," while in the post-surgery, they showed a greater body harmony and genital intimacy.

All this said, we know that patients of all ages report plausible information according to the interlocutor. For andrologists, the technique of the prosthetic implant, the absence of surgical complications, and the satisfaction of the patient and parents are important.

Case

My father was 40 when I was born. He was very kind and helpful. He never spanked me, although he didn't need to, his gaze was enough to keep you in line. But when I grew up a bit, maybe after 8 years, he started to be "weird," and I didn't understand why. He had problems with my older sister, Anna, a rebellious, wild, and unscrupulous girl. She brought home joints and then denied smoking. He didn't talk to me anymore, he had become different. It seemed that he no longer trusted me, he was no longer kind and helpful, he seemed far away.

(Giovanni, the patient)

I had John too late, and maybe I wasn't ready to live this anguish: for him and for me. When Katia, my wife, pointed out to me that he was missing a testicle, I felt like dying. We took him to various pediatricians and urologists, and although we were comforted that the damage could be remedied with a prosthesis, we were alone, Katia and I, to decide whether to intervene immediately or wait for adolescence. My father then made things worse by saying to me, "It would have been better if John had been missing a leg than missing a testicle..." Yes, but did he know about me and my suffering?

(Matteo, the father)

I was alone in caring for John when he was a child. He was an easy child to manage, he ate and he slept. Except that he seemed so different from the other children. Only one testicle, would he have been strange? Different? Without saying anything to Matteo, I went alone to his pediatrician. But he didn't convince me. I left the hospital more agitated than before. I saw another one and yet another. Then I said "enough!" and I spoke with Matteo. He told me he had already noticed this, one day while changing John on the changing table.

From that moment on, Matteo dedicated himself to Giovanni. He seemed confident in waiting for any surgery ... Then I had a miscarriage and so, without realizing it, Giovanni and I, we shared the tasks: I fell into depression, and Matteo made up for me, between one work commitment and another, taking care of Anna and Giovanni.

(Katia, the mother)

Travelling for work, I always thought about how different it would have been if I had had my mother by my side. She was always affectionate, calm, she took care of me and listened to me until I was 8, when she fell to the ground, not breathing. She would have told me what to decide for Giovanni.

And in the meantime the years passed, in the hope that a pediatrician would advise us when to have the surgery.

(Matteo)

At thirteen, Giovanni returned home after having had a fight with a school friend I asked him what had happened and why it had come to blows. He never told me why, but he shouted "I'm tired of feeling ashamed, of being half a boy. Why don't you and dad do something?, I'm deformed!"

Towards evening, I spoke to him from behind the door and I heard him crying.

(Katia)

Giovanni had decided for the whole family: he wanted to be a boy with a normal body, a boy like everyone else, a boy who "should not always be afraid of being found ugly, deformed, and abnormal"; these are the phrases used by Giovanni's parents at the first meeting with the psychosexologist.

Is it the boy who has to make this decision? Should we wait until his discomfort?

> Giovanni was ridiculous as a child, he always laughed for no reason. He was Dad's favourite. Mum was always with me. I often heard him crying at night because he felt ugly and strange.
>
> I was aware of my brother's one testicle, my mother often talked about it with Dad "When shall we do it?" he would often say, "And what if the operation fails....
>
> And I said to myself, "when will this torment end? Today, now that I am 18, I say to myself that I was a fool not to understand.
>
> (Anna, the sister)

Giovanni, now 13, has again been seen by an andrologist. The diagnostic procedure has deemed him suitable for testicular prosthesis intervention. He seems tense and anxious at the meeting with the surgeon, the psychosexologist, and his family members.

In front of the drawings made by the specialist, regarding the type of implant he will use, Giovanni appears attentive and shows no signs of hesitation about the surgical recommendation.

> *"Now that we are alone Giovanni"* begins the psychosexologist *"can you tell me what you are feeling?"*

"I'm really scared, I've never spoken to anyone about my problem."

Let us make the task easier.

> *Would you prefer to draw your body? It's easier to explain how you feel, what feelings do you have? You can say anything you want, even that I ask you too many questions.*

Giovanni takes pen and paper and draws a black pirate, with a black bandage on his left eye and a wooden leg.

> Well, this is me. I got into a fight for this at school, a friend of mine had drawn it for me, saying to all my companions "Giovanni, he's ugly like a pirate, who will ever have him?"

Giovanni felt exposed and

"I pounced on my classmate with such anger that I didn't even feel the punches I was taking. Another classmate split us up and took me home. He told me that he had never seen me so infuriated and that he didn't understand why I had taken him so seriously. That guy was a troublemaker with everyone. I should have known it. Yeah, but I was tired of hiding myself. The worst is that the fury also took me at home and in the evening I snapped. My father hugged me for a long time; he said nothing, and the next day, Mum told me that we had an appointment here in the hospital."

The andrological and pediatric surgical criterion follows orthodox lines of clinical and hospital experience, but sometimes the adolescent—former child—has many things to say that can affect subsequent surgical satisfaction and communication with medical staff.

Similarly, parents of young children have a great deal of responsibility for education, health, and well-being, which they cannot solve just by listening to the heart, they sometimes have to decide "urgently" or because their child is uncomfortable.

- "I felt my blood freeze when Giovanni shouted that evening", Matteo reports, in a second conversation with his wife Katia and the psychosexologist. "I felt irresponsible for not having acted before and for having thought that Giovanni would have enough strength to overcome everything sooner or later.
- I felt just like my father, an incapable parent. When my mother died, my father only had the courage to tell me 'put on a strong mask, because life goes on, and from now on, you have to do it alone.'"

When the psychosexologist points out to Matteo that at the age of 8, Giovanni had the feeling that he, Matteo, had also left

"I hadn't noticed, but Giovanni is right. I'm not certain, maybe just around when my son was that age, they diagnosed me with a form of multiple sclerosis, fortunately slow and not progressing. I felt that I would not see Giovanni and Anna grow up, and I closed in on myself."

During two preparatory meetings for the operation, Giovanni drew a series of maps of his body in the making: starting from the outline of the pirate, looking in the mirror, he modified his face, legs, and abdomen.

In agreement with the psychosexologist and the surgical team, he hung his drawings on the wall of the room for the short stay in hospital. To the nurses who asked him "what are those drawings?" Giovanni replied

"It's me, from ugly to beautiful."

Giovanni's parents also met the psychosexologist before and after their son's prosthetic intervention. Anna was given the freedom to be present at the talks or to write on a sheet what she wanted to say to the psychosexologist. At the beginning of the meeting with the parents, in the case of her absence, the content of her message would be read out and discussed with the parents.

Anna simply wrote

"I would like my parents not to be afraid to be happy."

In the pre- and post-surgical stages, Giovanni began to express perplexity about his future.

"If I have a girl, will she notice that I'm not entirely real?"

"What do you mean by 'not real'?" (psychosexologist)

"I have a prosthesis, will it have a strange feeling, like touching plastic?"

The question of whether or not to tell a partner in advance, of having a prosthesis, how the girl will react, still being able to have sexual intercourse, and feeling "the feelings of pleasure that all boys feel" are the silent dilemmas of many boys with monorchidism.

For the psychosexologist though, this passage means that we are over surgery, the trauma of the teenager's old feeling of diversity.

Giovanni, and those like him, begin to plan for the future, to feel "in a new condition as a normal boy" who must acquire new experiences. The surgeon also has a role in this phase. Who better than him, as a man, can validate what he has achieved with the psychosexologist?

13.2 Giovanni and His Family's Point of View

The case history of Giovanni shows that one cannot go through surgery without also knowing how much experience of disease has conditioned the physical, emotional, and relational growth of each individual.

Giovanni's father, marked by the loss of his mother, brought himself up with an emotionally absent father and then had a diagnosis of multiple sclerosis as an adult, sees his son's monorchidism as a "destiny that repeats itself."

First as a son and then as a father, he experienced loneliness, the fear of losing another family member, the inadequacy of his parental remit

"I was afraid not to see Giovanni and Anna as adults."

Katia, in her turn, is not able to overcome the feeling of inadequacy:

"I gave birth to three children. One is no longer here, Giovanni suffered so much, and Anna, so wild, perhaps suffered more than anyone else so that during my depression, it was she who gave me courage."

Giovanni "from pirate to sporty marathon boy" confessed to the psychosexologist how much anger the suffering of being different produces.

Anna, becoming a woman, wanted to leave an exclusive space to Giovanni in the surgical preparation

"because he deserves it. He has a right to see himself as he wants. I was lucky, I like myself. I didn't cry because I was missing a part of my femininity."

13.3 The Surgeon's Point of View

Clinical and psychosexological knowledge are complementary, and every professional is prepared for his or her role and to influence team knowledge.

Just as Giovanni's family understood how much strength there was in the unity of relationships and affections, so surgeon and psychosexologist choose each time how best to invest in the individual boy (and family system) to give clinical, emotional, relational answers.

13.4 Conclusions

Children, teenagers, and adults facing monorchidism feel committed to being part of the problem and the solution of the problem.

If the surgeon can offer technique, experience, empathy, scientific, and human knowledge, the psyche of individuals and the family history of the young patient are the prerequisites for building a therapeutic goal compatible with the feelings of all.

Including doctors and psychosexologists.

It is important to ask yourself as a specialist

How did I feel in the midst of this family?

and

How did this child/youth feel?

Our feeling as specialists is not without excessive mirroring, intolerance, or disharmony of character, compared to our clinical and biographical experience.

This is also part of the therapeutic process. A perfectly implanted prosthesis is not the only condition for patient and family satisfaction. Especially if it is not accompanied by listening, acceptance, and a therapeutic relationship built on the emotional and relational needs of all participants.

Patient compliance? It is an ongoing process, not an objective achieved with perfect surgery. Especially in the case of children and adolescents.

Their growth, their feelings, their experiences of intimacy, and their relationships will be the true cornerstones of a therapeutic process started many years before.

13.5 Sample Self-Assessment for the Andrologist

This is not a test and no structured answers are expected. This is a way to learn and improve our clinical-therapeutic style.

If you had been Giovanni's surgeon:

1. Would you have immediately empathized with the boy?
2. Would you have excluded the parents and the sister from further interviews?
3. Would you have asked yourself "what's the point" of knowing the family history?
4. Would you have acted differently to the way described?
5. Do you feel more comfortable with the mothers or with the fathers of the children visiting your outpatient clinic?
6. Would you use a psychosexologist to understand whether in some cases you identify too much with your patients?
7. How competent do you feel in prosthetic surgical techniques?
8. How much attention do you pay to "your patients minds"?
9. If the psychosexologist told you "This family needs to 'recover' from too many family diagnoses and bereavements. Be paternal and empathetic with everyone except Giovanni. What would it mean to you?

10. If the psychosexologist told you to: "Agree with Giovanni to observe the outcome of the surgery together in hospital. Bring the drawing that he made in the first interview and compare it with the final body map that the boy hung on the wall of the room. What would this mean for you?
11. If the psychosexologist told you to: "Suggest to Giovanni that he write down, in the first weeks after surgery, all his physical sensations connected to the testicular prosthesis and to his emotions. ..." What would be the meaning of this instruction for you?
12. Would you agree with Giovanni on a long-term follow-up? What type? With the parents?

13.6 Sample Questionnaire for Medical History Evaluation

Proposed by the psychosexologist to the patient and his parents.

For the parents:

1. Before turning to this department, how did you try to solve Giovanni's problem?
2. When, in your opinion, did Giovanni become aware of his monorchidism?
3. How has Giovanni's attitude toward his body changed, if it has changed, over time? Does he lock himself in the bathroom, undress in his room alone?
4. What attitude has Giovanni shown toward your physicality and that of his sister? Does he embrace you, is he physical in his gestures, or does he avoid touching and being touched?
5. When was the first time that Giovanni washed himself, in his intimate areas, without your help?
6. Is your bedroom door usually open or closed?

For the patient (Giovanni):

1. Who knows you are here, in hospital today?
2. What did you think about on the way here?
3. What is your expectation of the surgeon's work?
4. Does it feel strange, talking to a psychosexologist?
5. What idea have you had so far of the doctors and people who will help you in this process?
6. Are you worried for your parents?
7. If your sister were here, would you be embarrassed to speak in front of her?
8. If the implant goes well but you do not like the look of it, what would be your reaction?

For siblings (Giovanni's sister):

1. Are you worried for Giovanni?
2. What makes you most anxious about the post-surgical process?
3. Whom have you talked to about this?
4. If you had a boyfriend, would you talk to him about it?
5. How do you think you will treat Giovanni after the operation? Will you give him a hug? Will you make a joke?
6. Have you spoken to your parents about your thoughts and worries??
7. Which of your parents do you think is the less ready to face this experience? Why?

References

1. Kogan S (2014) The clinical utility of testicular prosthesis placement in children with genital and testicular disorders. Transl Androl Urol 3(4):391–397
2. Turek PJ, Master VA (2004) Testicular Prosthesis Study Group: safety and effectiveness of a new saline filled testicular prosthesis. J Urol 172:1427–1430

3. Adshead J, Khoubehi B, Wood J, Rustin G (2003) Testicular implants and patient satisfaction: a questionnaire-based study of men after orchidectomy for testicular cancer. BJU Int 88:559–562
4. Bodiwala D, Summerton DJ, Terry TR (2007) Testicular prostheses: development and modern usage. Ann R Coll Surg Engl 89:349–353
5. Ferro F, Caterino S, Lais A (1991) Testicular prosthesis in children: a simplified insertion technique. Eur Urol 19(3):230–232
6. Libman JL, Pippi-Salle JL, Chan PTK (2006) The use of a suprascrotal or "wink" incision for placing a testicular prosthesis. BJU Int 98:1051–1053
7. Ferro F, Borrelli P, Lucchetti MC (2004) A surgical method to preserve testicular function and to restore cosmetic appearance in hypogonadal men. J Urol 171:2368–2370
8. Adshead J et al (2001) Testicular implants and patient satisfaction: a study based on a questionnaire of men after orchiectomy for testicular cancer. BJU Int 88:559–562
9. Peycelon M et al (2016) Testicular prosthesis in children: you better before? J Pediatr Urol 12(4):237–239
10. Elder JS et al (1989) Testicular prosthesis childish. J Urol 141(6):1413–1415
11. Weissbach L et al (1979) Testicular prosthesis implantation: psychological aspects. J Urol 18(3):151–156

Sperm Retrieval in the Azoospermic Patient in Young Adult and Humans: The Klinefelter Syndrome

14

Elena Vittoria Longhi and Alessandro Franceschelli

14.1 Introduction

The techniques of retrieval of testicular sperm, associated with the intracytoplasmic injection of sperm, have changed the field of treatment of male infertility and have made fatherhood possible (impossible until 20 years ago) for azoospermic men.

Clinical aspects of sperm retrieval include the etiology of infertility, the age, and the testicular volume of the patient (Schema 14.1).

For nonobstructive azoospermia these three criteria can be considered alone or combined with endocrinological data. The literature offers data *on cryptorchidism, varicocele, and Klinefelter syndrome.*

Cryptorchidism is one of the most common infantile malformations and affects 3% of term newborn males. This condition is related to male infertility, testicular tumors, testicular torsion, and inguinal hernias [1]. Studies on clinical factors related to sperm retrieval in patients with cryptorchidism have considered limited statistics, and the conclusions remain controversial. Raman and Schlegel [2], in a study of 38 azoospermal men, found correlations between sperm retrieval rate and age following orchidopessia.

Patients who had undergone surgery before the age of 10 had a better sperm retrieval rate than men who underwent orchidopessia at 10 years or older.

While more recently Wiser A. [3], studying 40 patients undergoing orchidopessia and presenting azoospermia, found no significant differences between men undergoing surgery before or after 10 years of age. *Varicocele* is an important male infertility factor with a high incidence. It seems that the benefits of surgical treatment in terms of sperm quality are hard to question, but the problem becomes complex for patients with azoospermia associated with varicocele who wish to conceive naturally after surgical correction [4].

Many studies have evaluated whether the effectiveness of surgical treatment of varicocele prior to TESE improves the chances of sperm recovery.

E. V. Longhi et al., *Psychosexual Counseling in Andrological Surgery*,
https://doi.org/10.1007/978-3-319-99646-2_14

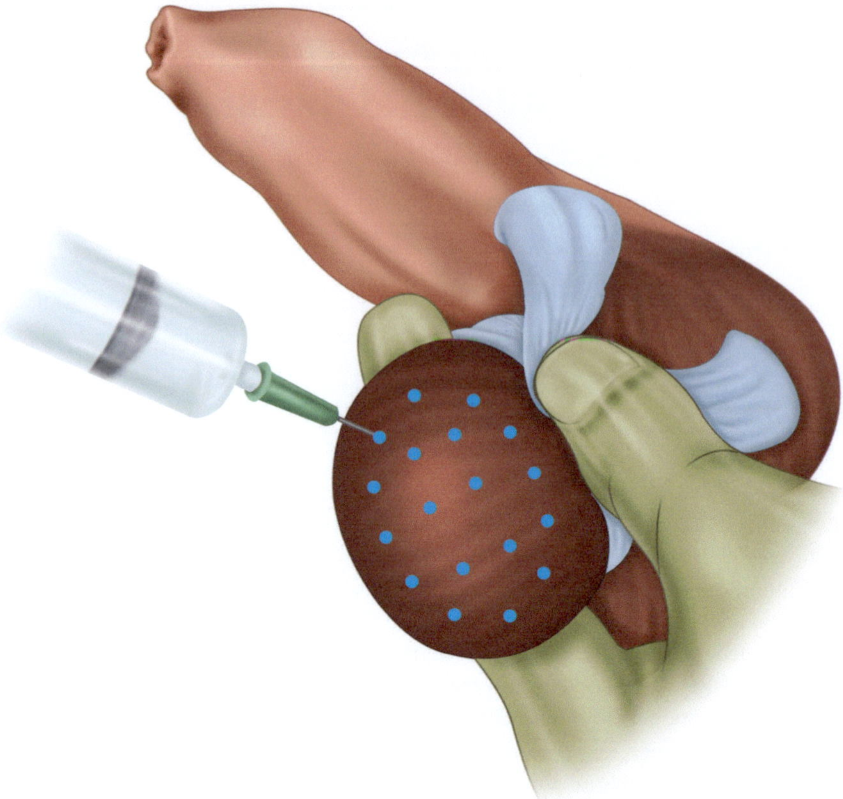

Schema 14.1 A schematic drawing of the mapping of the FNA which shows the "bandage" gauze testicle for fixation and the sampling pattern marked on the scrotum 8 (adapted with permission). Fine needle aspiration Fna

Ninety-six patients with varicocele and nonobstructive azoospermia were studied: 66 men had undergone previous surgical treatment for varicocele at least 5 months previously, and 30 patients had not previously been treated. The average age of the men studied, testicular volumes, FSH levels, and partner ages were not significantly different in the two groups.

The results showed a better retrieval rate for the treated group—53% compared to 30%—but there were no significant differences in embryo quality, implantation rates, and miscarriage variables.

14.2 Evaluation of Azoospermic Patients

Initial evaluation of azoospermic patients includes a complete medical history (such as previous surgery, cryptorchidism, history of malignancy, systemic diseases) and physical examination.

Small or atrophic testes are highly suggestive of NOA, while normal testicular volume, enlargement of the epididymis, and absence of the vas deference are indicative of OA

Semen analysis can help to distinguish between OA and NOA, for example, low ejaculate volume gives evidence of an obstructive form, as well as low fructose and low pH.

Hormonal evaluation (FSH, LH, and testosterone levels) is recommended, and finding of elevated FSH level associated with normal semen volume is diagnostic of NOA.

Scrotum ultrasound must be done for the study of the testis and epididymis, while transrectal ultrasound must be performed in the presence of low ejaculate volume.

Karyotype and chromosome Y microdeletions testing must be done when NOA is suspected, while mutations of the cystic fibrosis transmembrane regulator (CFTR) protein in cases of OA (6).

14.3 Treatment

14.3.1 Obstructive Azoospermia

In cases of obstruction of the seminal ducts and in the presence of normal spermatogenesis, confirmed by histology, microsurgical epididymovasostomy (epididymal obstruction) or a vasovasostomy (vas deferens obstruction) is indicated. Outcomes of microsurgical reconstruction have improved over the past four decades and currently include 70–99.5% patency/36–92% pregnancy rates for VV and 30–90% patency/20–50% pregnancy rates for VE.19–21 (DA SPMG 2818).

In cases of congenital obstruction due to agenesia of the vas deferens or of the epididymis, microsurgical epididymal sperm aspiration (MESA) or sperm extraction from the testis (testicular sperm extraction—TESE) in combination with assisted fertilization (ICSI, intracytoplasmic sperm injection) is the treatment of choice (7).

14.3.2 Nonobstructive Azoospermia

For patients affected by NOA, the only chance of treatment is surgical sperm retrieval. For many years the standard treatment has been represented by conventional single or multiple TESE.

TESE has an average retrieval rate around 50% in NOA men. Possible complications are low but include loss of significant amount of testicular tissue in patients that already have small testis, hematoma, and devascularization (8). In recent years, after his first description by Schelegel in 1999, this surgical technique has been widely used. The testis is opened widely in an equatorial plane along the mid portion. And using magnification of an operating microscope (20–25×). It is possible to clearly visualized dilated and more opaque tubules in which the probability of retrieval sperm is higher.

Several studies have shown how microTESE allows for greater chance of retrieving sperm and lower removal of testicular tissue compared to conventional TESE.

1. Evaluation of the azoospermic male. Oates R. Asian Journal of Andrology (2012) 14, 82–87
2. EAU Guidelines on male infertility
3. Male infertility: Pathogenesis and clinical diagnosis. C. Krausz. Best Practice & Research Clinical Endocrinology & Metabolism 25 (2011) 271–285
4. The genetic causes of male factor infertility: a review. O'Flynn, O'Brien KL, Varghese AC, Agarwal A. Fertil Steril. 2010 Jan;93(1):1–12
5. Klinefelter syndrome A.M. Wikström, 240 L. Dunkel/Best Practice & Research Clinical Endocrinology & Metabolism 25 (2011) 239–250
6. Review of Azoospermia Wosnitzer M, Goldstein M, Hardy MP. Spermatogenesis. 2014
7. Obstructive azoospermia: reconstructive techniques and results. Baker K, Sabanegh Jr E. Clinics (Sao Paulo). 2013;68 Suppl 1:61–73
8. Outcome of microdissection TESE compared with conventional TESE in nonobstructive azoospermia: a systematic review. Deruyver Y, Vanderschueren D, Van der Aa F. Andrology. 2014 Jan;2(1):20–4
9. Comparison of microdissection testicular sperm extraction, conventional testicular sperm extraction, and testicular sperm aspiration for nonobstructive azoospermia: a systematic review and meta-analysis. Bernie AM, Mata DA, Ramasamy R, Schlegel PN. Fertil Steril. 2015 Nov;104(5):1099–103

The Case

Fulvio (29, pharmacist) and Marta (31, employee) are sent by the andrologist surgeon to a meeting with the psychosexologist to evaluate the emotional state and the relationship of the couple. Fulvio has already been treated surgically for varicocele and has now discovered that he is azoospermic. He is on a waiting list for sperm retrieval. *For the andrologist, he is the most fragile figure of the couple*

14.4 The Interview with the Couple

(Psychosexologist) What did you think when the surgeon invited you to this introductory conversation with me?

"In this difficult situation" begins Marta "Someone has to help us out. Frankly I don't blame Fulvio and in fact I admire his courage in undergoing these procedures but the anxiety of not being able to have a child has become unbearable for us."

(Psychosexologist) *Do you see yourself in your wife's description Fulvio?*

"*We are not married doctor.*" Fulvio answers "*We have lived together for 2 years. Or rather, I went to live at Marta's, because she had the larger house. Of course, the situation is not easy, you can understand. The problem is that this whole situation is much bigger than we are and I wonder where it will take us!*"

Marta and Fulvio have known each other for 3 years, and they live together out of love and choice and the sincere desire to build a family. Both are very busy in their professional lives: Fulvio works the night shifts in a pharmacy in the city center several days a week, and the rest of the time, he helps his father in his small pharmacy in the provinces.

Marta is a high-level employee and hopes soon to be promoted to a more important role.

At the age of 22, Marta underwent gynaecological surgery for endometriosis. And from that moment on, her sexuality seems to have weakened....

"All the care, attention and consideration have always been for me since I met Fulvio" continues Marta "He is very affectionate and helpful, always ready to fulfil my every desire ...... and suddenly I find myself giving courage to him, for something that should be natural ...... We always have to struggle ... even to have a child. I didn't think he would be weak too...."

"The thing is Doctor," intervenes Fulvio " that Marta has a self-centered character. She lives in her world and is not used to taking care of others. She's a generous, intelligent girl, full of interests, but it's the men in her home who are the 'top of the class'..."

Marta's father is in fact a judge of the Civil Court and by character "remains a judge inside and outside the house" says Marta "so my sister and I have learned to say yes to him.... Also because my mother is too indulgent with him..."

<u>These first descriptions show how the surgical treatment proposed to Fulvio has revealed generalized anxieties related to man-woman relations, power relations in the two-party relationship, and insensitivity and inadequacy toward the solution of problems related to intimacy.</u>

> *<u>What does all this have to do with surgery?</u>* If the couple were not supportive and complementary in this stressful clinical process, surely the outcome of the surgical procedure could also become a "new battlefield." It could further undermine Fulvio's virility ..... putting at a distance the possibility of having a child and compromising the couple's alliance in future projects.

Sometimes, Marta resumes, "I have the feeling that Fulvio is contrary just to make me anxious....He doesn't speak at home, he only smiles in the pharmacy... He looks sad, worried and if I ask him "What's wrong?" He answers "nothing, I just have a great sense of guilt"....

- Usually azoospermia in a young man involves a great sense of frustration, while undergoing surgical procedures in order to "prove oneself virile" adds shame, pain, sexual incapacity, and a great deal of anger.
- This is often aimed at himself because of fear of "losing the partner."

"In recent months, the tension between us has increased," Fulvio resumes. "In the pharmacy, I am ironical and smile because I have to hide this situation. Then I hear the criticism of my father-in-law, he looks at me with compassion and sexual relations with Martha haven't existed for months. I don't have any desire, I don't have any spontaneous erections and I don't know how to keep the pieces together......"

To Keep in Mind 1

The sexual nature of this relationship had never been a "great deal." Marta's endometriosis and severe pelvic pain before gynaecological surgery had been a severe limitation of intimacy. Then, who knows why, the "ghost" pains seemed to persist.

"Often Marta said to me 'don't touch me'" Fulvio describes "and I learned, out of respect and because I saw her suffering, to limit physical contact. Then, I realized that we are no longer intimate..."

Fulvio admits to having suffered from this lack of physical contact and to having noticed Marta being intolerant, sometimes contemptuous, "You're good for nothing," he seems to have been told in a moment of discouragement, after his attempt to embrace and kiss her.

The picture begins to emerge. This umpteenth clinical trial for the couple has definitely put Fulvio in a corner, and the psychosexologist's hypothesis is that Marta's sudden desire to have a son, "is also a way to see if Fulvio is up to the job," at least as a father.....

Subsequent questions from the psychosexologist's interview verify this hypothesis. "I've never been so taken with sex" confesses Marta "and I thought that having a son would give me the chance with Fulvio to give a different meaning to my life as a woman...."

It is clear that Marta *confuses sexuality with fertility* so the psychosexologist deals with this issue as a couple, and Fulvio, after a while, appears more relaxed.

"It's strange (the psychosexologist). I have the feeling you seem more relaxed, especially you Fulvio ... Possibly (Fulvio) because what you said has clarified many things. It's not my fault that I was first diagnosed with varicocele and then with azoospermia. See Marta? I'm not a good for nothing... I'm just a clinically unlucky man... not a second class man...."

14.5 Sexological Notes

The anxious symmetry of this couple is channelled into the second and third successive meetings with the psychosexologist in a contract of complicity for two, based on:

1. *On a new way of experiencing sexuality*. An intimacy of an adult couple made of play and complicity and not only of sexual intercourse with coitus: a daily sexuality that gives back to Fulvio and Marta a means to eliminate the stress of performance at all costs: taking a shower together, undressing one another to prepare for bed in the evening,.
2. *On a new way of planning "parenthood"* A process in which the couple did NOT have to channel all expectations of the future of the couple. Almost as if saying "either parents or no sex, no intimacy as a couple."
3. *About a relationship that will help accompany Fulvio to the planned surgery.* A relationship that is more complicit in tackling and resolving the problem together. Where each individual would play an equal role (50%) and not a relationship sometimes between parent/daughter, parent/son.
4. *On a varied surgical post-surgery full of projects for the couple and not only aimed at parenting*. "You owe me a grandson" was the sentence the father-in-law handed down to Fulvio, and the couple had "emotionally regressed to do their duty to silence the judge."

The psychosexologist and the couple, independently of one another, forward reports of their interview to the surgeon.

On the day of the sperm retrieval, Fulvio's mother introduced herself: "my husband couldn't find a substitute in the pharmacy but is still ready to come in the event of an emergency," she told me.

She appeared an elegant, calm, quiet woman, with great esteem for her pharmacist son and great apprehension "because you understand, doctor... an operation is always an operation..."

And then:

"My son told me that he feels very supported here, because he feels understood...... For a mother and a father this is very important. Fulvio has so much pain inside...he was afraid that Martha would leave him...and that he would be very ill... He and his father are proud, good, transparent people, but with an iron will..."

- Speaking with the woman, the psychosexologist sensed that, unlike Marta's family, in which a pyramidal hierarchy existed, in Fulvio's family, father and mother were, as he himself said, "like two peas in a pod."
- An allied couple, a couple sometimes with different ideas, but with a strong basic emotional bond and a strong loyalty to each other.

"I understood when talking to your mother how much effort she made to withstand Marta's competitive style," the psychosexologist told Fulvio and Marta in the first post-surgical meeting. "And how difficult it was for Marta to accept a man who did not impose rules, but sought rules with her...."

These considerations served both to establish that neither one had any more power nor the conviction to impose it. And that the future son could not be the "third" who could tell them, after the judge, how "to behave and to support each other..."

14.6 What Are the Motives of the Couple?

Too much psychology? If we do not work on the relationships of a couple, on the balances of each, and on the idea of a couple that each brings from their own family of origin, how is it possible to build projects in the making? Dealing with such a delicate surgery?

One is a parent before the child is born, and it is necessary to define the boundaries between one's role as a child and one's role as a partner/lover, so as not to project one's own biography onto the unborn child.

The surgeon is responsible for retrieving seminal fluid, not the affective maturity and awareness of the virility of each individual patient.

The psychosexologist works to create balances and activate processes of life already existent within the couple but unconscious in both Fulvio and Marta until the moment of confrontation with a clinical event which was too delicate for two souls who were only looking for "acceptance" from each other.

14.7 No More Rare Disease

Klinefelter syndrome is a karyotype disorder that results from a supernumerary X chromosome and can be expressed in two forms: mosaic and non-mosaic.

This not uncommon condition (it affects 1 in 600 men) is usually associated with infertility.

Today the sperm retrieval rate in patients with Klinefelter is about 50% [5].

Previous literature suggested that age and testicular volume were prognostic factors, but a more recent study showed no correlation between clinical parameters and sperm retrieval [6].

However, these studies focused on a small number of patients between the ages of 20 and 51.

The review of 13 articles on 373 Klinefelter patients with azoospermia who underwent sperm collection showed that clinical parameters were not a satisfactory prognostic factor.

14.8 Clinical Practice

Thus far, research and scientific literature. *Now, daily clinical practice:*

What kind of patients are we dealing with?

Klinefelter patients (KS) show high stature, small testicles, gynecomastia in late puberty, wide hips, sparse body hair, signs of androgen deficiency, and low serum testosterone, alongside elevated gonadotropins, azoospermia, and oligospermia with hyalinization and seminiferous tubular fibrosis [7].

Adolescence represents for KS patients a moment of reinvestment and redefinition of the relationship with parents and medical figures with reference to the management of the syndrome.

The need for independence and the search for autonomy (often confused with anarchy or opposition, as with all processes of adolescent growth) have a significant influence on the patient's expectations when dealing with adults.

The focal point seems to be the awareness and perception of one's own body:

The boy with KS needs, more so than his peers, to compare himself, to elaborate, and to overcome the emotional and social difficulties deriving from the comparison with "normal" bodies. Think, for example, how much anxiety, shame, and otherness gynecomastia can cause.

And what of sexuality?

Although psychosexual behavior is in most cases male, erectile dysfunction and premature ejaculation (as with moderate libido reduction) produce generalized anxiety, guilt, otherness, introversion, and, in more serious cases, self-destructive and devaluing thoughts.

A study by Raboch [8] showed that 86% of Ks participants were married, and the average age of falling in love was much older than in the control group.

An earlier study [9] studied the sexual development and activity of men with somatic development disorders.

14.9 HTDM and SAM Questionnaires

These patient groups were studied (with HTDM and SAM questionnaires):

1. The control group consisted of 345 married men from infertile marriages, who were adequately developed somatically and had normozoospermia in ejaculate and good potency.
2. 48 unilateral cryptorchids and 57 adult bilateral cryptorchids.
3. In 101 married men with distinct testicular hypoplasia, the long axis of each sex gland was shorter than 30 mm.
4. 110 patients had Klinefelter's syndrome.

While delay in heterosexual development was found in only two groups (groups 3 and 4), clearly reduced activity in sexual life was found in all four pathological samples.

And then there is the psychopathological risk. Each KS child experiences limited school success, emotional and behavioral difficulties, and dysfunctional family relationships, often with psychotic-type communication.

How crucial life experiences, e.g., when confronted with derision from peers (onset of anxiety and mood disorders), with aggression and relationships of abandonment or disqualification and marginalization by the peer group are for the development of psychic disorders in the KS boy were stressed.

A study based on the use of DSM-IV-TR (*Diagnostic and Statistical Manual of Mental Disorders*) estimated the prevalence of mental disorders in a sample of 51 boys—average age 12.2 years—suffering from Klinefelter's syndrome [10]:

1. 65% of the sample had learning difficulties
2. 63% had ADHD
3. 24% had depressive disorders
4. 8% suffered from psychosis
5. 2% suffered from schizophrenia

To Keep in Mind 2

The intellectual level of boys and men with KS is on average lower, especially with regard to verbal IQ. However, the real problem is that these cognitive dysfunctions in the areas of language, executive functioning, and social interaction often worsen if not continuously monitored.

On average, boys and men with KS are at risk in relation to social adjustment and interactions with others.

1. *Psychosexual psychologists are therefore confronted with extremely complex patients with latent vulnerability. They show: extreme shyness, awkward and short-term interaction, extensive social apathy, difficulty in relating to peers, generalized anxiety syndrome, and social phobia. Some studies* [11] *describe KS boys as calm, reflective, and not very assertive.*
2. They are patients who must be followed throughout their lives and who have to be treated with testosterone in case of hypogonadism.
3. Not always diagnosed at gestation, if diagnosed later in life, they exhibit physical and emotional suffering and social distress. It is still not known how many patients do not seek medical consultations or specific treatment, due to apathy, negligence, or lack of information.

4. The impact of KS during the life of the fetus and the initial period after birth remains an open question. Only 25% of patients are diagnosed before puberty.
5. *Psychological support for the child and parents or for the adult is often underestimated* and left to the decision of the individual and the family. Many parents do not know how to deal with the sexual development of their children and their often avoidant behavior, and endocrinologists do not often recognize these needs, if not made explicit by patients or the family.
6. Psychological support would foster doctor-patient communication and compliance with therapies and surgical treatments, as well as better social integration and a relational ability which is more versatile and less constrained by anxiety-phobic-depressive syndrome.
7. Not to exclude, their rarity notwithstanding, cases of suicide or progressive autism, which are much more frequent in adolescents and young adults.

The therapeutic proposal—The need for *an integrated and multidisciplinary therapeutic proposal on three levels* even seems superfluous:

1. *Psychological support*—Should be aimed at restoring the patient's motivation, hope, and capacity for integration and at building his own future. It is precisely for this reason that it should start early, so as to influence the child's (and future adult's) level of self-esteem and to overcome anxieties, insecurities, and phobias. With the appropriate involvement of the parents, informing them about the various clinical, emotional, and sexual stages of the pathology in the process of bringing up the child/youth
2. *Educational project*—Should be structured to facilitate the acquisition of the different stages of language learning, reduce the lack of attention on the frontline of executive skills, progressively increase school performance, and counter any motor difficulties. As well as encouraging the KS child/youth to practice a sport, to improve physical skills, and encourage interaction with peers
3. *Psychotherapy project*—This would include the use, when necessary, of psychopharmacology, individual therapy for the child/man and/or family member in the presence of dysfunctional and psychotic communication styles

To Keep in Mind 3

How can the techniques of testicular sperm recovery be reconciled with the complex and vulnerable personality of these KS patients?

Young people and adults with Klinefelter syndrome also show great difficulty in identifying the emotions of others on the basis of facial expressions, emotional tone of the voice, direction of the gaze, and nonverbal communication.

As a result, KS children and adults seem to show higher degrees of suffering during the very frequent clinical checks and even experience deep anguish if they feel they are the object of slight criticism.

The limited emotional capacity (as a consequence of neurocognitive dysfunctions) then limits these patients in physiological response, in the expression of feelings and in the organization of action [12].

Young people and adults with KS, when subjected to the screening of emotive video clips, highlighted difficulties in identifying with the main character, in giving a name to feelings and sensations aroused by the plot, and in assessing their emotional state in accordance with the protagonist and other actors.

Poor regulation of emotions was associated with lower quality friendships, reduced interpersonal sensitivity, asocial tendencies, and greater friction between young people [13–15].

There is no doubt that in the presence of such complex patients, surgery is the tip of an iceberg which cannot be ignored or taken for granted.

Every patient will bring with him, in addition to the desire for fatherhood, areas of relational and emotional growth which have not always been explored and which cannot fail to combine with the stressful impact of these clinical practices at the expense of success and of becoming yet another source of "otherness, exclusion, and shame."

Turning to a psychosexologist is also a way to make the patient aware of any unconfirmed personal issues or sources of insecurity: in addition to giving him the possibility to place clinical practices in a supported, defined, and conscious emotional and relational context. Probably successfully.

14.10 Conclusions

Certainly clinical practices have, over time, realized the objectives of fertility and parenthood, which otherwise would have been excluded, not for lack of will but due to their impossibility.

Human complexity, as adaptable and powerful as it may be, is not always correlated with natural and painless growth processes.

The psychosexological evaluation of such patients is the premise for understanding the boy/man and facilitating his plans, his future growth, his virility, and his confidence in his role.

The preparation of a clinical-therapeutic team also involves a continuous self-learning by individual specialists who cannot ignore the peculiarity of the patient and their expectations of success.

14.11 Returning to the Case

14.11.1 Self-Check Path

As always, there are no right or wrong answers. This is just a way to confront our therapeutic style and sensitivity.

1. How much do you rely on your clinical experience and how much do you share emotional and behavioral aspects of the patient with your colleagues?
2. When facing a Klinefelter's boy, how much do you value the interaction with his parents, as well as with the boy?
3. Is the surgical practice of testicular sperm retrieval merely a clinical practice?
4. How clear is the distinction between virility and fertility for the patient? Do you check this with the patient and the couple?
5. If a patient who has already been surgically treated for varicocele comes to you for a consultation and, in your opinion, the operation does not seem to have been carried out with orthodoxy, do you criticize your colleague? Do you seek possible mediation with the patient's requests?
6. If an adult Klinefelter's patient experiences difficulties in the continuity of therapy, how do you deal with the problem?

If you find that the psychological aspects of a patient are multiple and complex, do you (a) send him/her to the psychosexologist? (b) seek to deal with the therapeutic methodology with the help of colleagues? (c) feel you are wasting time?

14.11.2 Medical History Questions

14.11.2.1 For the Couple

- How have you dealt with the situation so far? Have you been challenged, have you had cause for conflict, and have you left the problem to the specialists?
- If it is not possible to conceive a child, have you considered other opportunities?
- Who among your acquaintances or relatives is acquainted with the situation?
- What expectations do you have as to the outcome of these surgical and clinical practices?
- How have you addressed the issue of sexuality during this period?
- When were you diagnosed with Klinefelter's syndrome?
- Do you feel that you are well followed clinically and psychologically?
- If you are not talking about your illness, what interests do you discuss with friends and relatives and with your partner?

14.11.2.2 For the Parents of Young Klinefelter's Patients

- Since your child was diagnosed with KS, how has your life as a couple and as parents changed?
- What difficulties do you encounter with the families of other healthy children?
- How have you so far tried to overcome your child's character and relationship problems?
- When clinical checkups approach, how does your child's mood change (if at all)?
- What would you ask of your doctors to make you feel less alone in the management of your child?
- Has the diagnosis of your child's KS changed your relationship as a couple?
- Do you have or would you have liked other children?

References

1. Garrone G et al (2010) Distopias Testiculares e Malformacoes Genitais, Urologia Fundamental. Plamark, San Paulo, pp 383–389
2. Raman JD et al (2003) Testicular sperm extraction with intracytoplasmic sperm injection is effective for the treatment of non-obstructive azoospermia associated with cryptorchidism. J Urol 170(4):1287–1290
3. Wiser A et al (2009) Age the incidence of testicular sperm extraction results orchidopessia. Reprod Online Biomed 19(6):778–783
4. Baazeem A et al (2011) Varicocele and male factor infertility treatment: a new meta-analysis and review of the role of varicocele repair. Eur Urol 60(4):796–808
5. Madgar I et al (2002) Prognostic value of clinical and laboratory assessment with Klinefelter's syndrome not assisted reproductive therapy receive melosa. Fertil Steril 77(6):1167–1169
6. Koga M et al (2007) Clinical comparison of testicular sperm extraction succeeded and failed in patients with Klinefelter's syndrome not melosa. J Urol 70(2):341–345
7. Groth KA et al (2013) Clinical review: Klinefelter syndrome: a clinical update. J Clin Endocrinol Metab 98(1):20–30
8. Raboch J et al (2003) Serum testosterone levels and coital activity in men with somatosexual disorders. Neuro Endocrinol Lett 24:321–324
9. Raboch J et al (1979) Sexual development and somatic activity of men with developmental disabilities. J Androl 11(4):263–271
10. Boks MP et al (2007) Psychiatric morbidity and X chromosomal origin in Klinefelter sample. Schizophr Res 93:399–402
11. Visootsak J et al (2006) Klinefelter syndrome and other sex chromosomal aneuploidies. Orphanet J Rare Dis 1:42
12. Gyurak A et al (2011) Explicit and implicit emotional regulation: a dual-process structure. Cognit Emot 25:400–412
13. Lopes PN et al (2004) Emotional intelligence and social interaction. Pers Soc Psychol Bull 30:1018–1034
14. Lopes PN et al (2005) Ability of emotional regulation and quality of social interaction. Emotion 5:113–118
15. Pinkham AE et al (2006) Predictive social interpersonal skills and neurocognitive in schizophrenia. Res Psychiatry 143:167–178

Part III

The Patient and the Partner

Penile Prosthesis Implant in Neurological Patients

15

Elena Vittoria Longhi and Leonardo Misuraca

15.1 Introduction

Erectile dysfunction in patients affected by neurological disorders has many causes; neurological diseases affecting the cerebrum, brain stem, spinal cord, spinal roots, or peripheral nerves can alter sexual function because of a direct damage to the nerve pathways that allow sexual function Moreover sexual dysfunction can be a consequence of disability caused by poor bladder and bowel control, fatigue, muscle weakness, spasticity, immobility, tremor, cognitive impairment, and sensory problems.

Neurological patients present difficulty achieving and/or maintaining a valid erection, associated with a great variety of symptoms including decreased or loss in libido, painful or uncomfortable genital sensations (burning, tingling, numbness), altered orgasmic response, and ejaculatory dysfunction.

After the launch, in 1998, of sildenafil, many neurological patients have benefited of this treatment for erectile dysfunction. Today PDE5 inhibitors represent first-line treatment for erectile dysfunction for neurogenic patients, particularly those with spinal cord injury. Similar results can be obtained in patients with Parkinson's disease and multiple sclerosis, while in neurological diseases, such as epilepsy, data seems to suggest avoiding the use of PDE5Is as a first-line treatment for neurogenic ED due to possible severe adverse events [1].

When neurological patients do not respond to PDE5Is or to other treatment such as intracavernous injection of vasoactive drugs, penile implant remains the only possibility. The choice of which penile prosthesis should be implanted is conditioned by general and neurological conditions, because many patient have limited physical activity and hand movement.

In literature two studies report results of penile implant in neurological patients. In the first one, more than 200 patients underwent to the procedure, both hydraulic and semirigid implant: with a mean follow-up of 7 years, more than 80% of the patients declared to be satisfied with the implant. The overall complication rate was

E. V. Longhi et al., *Psychosexual Counseling in Andrological Surgery*,
https://doi.org/10.1007/978-3-319-99646-2_15

very low, 5%. The infection rate decreased from an initial 5.8 to 4.0% after the introduction of a change in antibiotic prophylaxis and the use of whole body disinfection. They observed a higher perforation rate with semirigid (18%) rather than with hydraulic prosthesis [2].

In the second one (3) has been evaluated the results of malleable penile implants in patients with spinal cord injury. Seventy-nine percent declare to be very satisfied or satisfied with the implant with an infection and erosion rate, respectively, of 8.3% and 4.2%.

15.2 Sexual Aspects

Sexuality is an important aspect of an individual's quality of life, and, not least of all, patients with neurological diseases put psychological and sexual well-being before other priorities of physical functionality.

A 2015 study Smith et al. [1] looked at patients between 46 and 67 years of age diagnosed with muscular dystrophy (MD), spinal cord injury (SCI), or post-polio syndrome (PPS). The participants responded to a qualitative questionnaire that included items such as:

1. Sexual satisfaction
2. The ability to have a satisfactory orgasm
3. The ability to achieve and maintain an erection

The use of pharmacological aids, vacuum devices, and penile prostheses was also evaluated.

The severity of the symptom was associated with the presence of problematic health conditions such as *depressive symptoms, pain interference, fatigue and anxiety, spasticity, and weakness in the lower extremities.*

The results showed that SCI patients reported better sexual function than other groups, with good orgasmic capacity, whereas men with MD reported "not having tried to achieve an erection" compared to 0% of individuals with PPS.

> Sexual satisfaction was strongly associated with sexual function for all patients (erectile function, quality and duration of erection, orgasmic capacity).

15.3 The Literature and the Clinical Practice

With regard to the efficacy of the aids adopted (*pharmacological, vacuum device, and penile prostheses*), MD patients reported the lowest satisfaction rate, with a small percentage indicating "sufficient" in the satisfaction range of sexual activity. Only 6% reported using the vacuum device and 1% implanted a penile prosthesis (SCI in particular).

There is no doubt that patients with SCI indicate sexual function as the first index for the recovery of physical and psychological function.

Khak et al. [3] studied 37 male veterans with hospitalization SCI for routine follow-up, who were given the GHQ-12 (Euro Quality of Life and General Health Questionnaire). The average age of the participants was 45.7 years with a duration of injury of 24 years.

All patients reported erectile dysfunction (ED) and 27% suffered from severe ED. Sleep deprivation and hypertension contributed to the progressive worsening of the dysfunction.

Furthermore: Cobo Cuenca et al. [4] investigated not only sexual dysfunction in patients with SCI but also self-esteem, quality of life, and anxiety levels.

Of patients with SCI, 89.4% showed erectile dysfunction, and 75.2% reported anejaculation. 16.47% showed signs of depression, and 35% showed anxiety. These were associated with further anxiety about social interaction, prospects for the future, and long-term affective-sexual capacity with a partner.

Although a penile prosthesis implant can restore a balance between the desire for satisfactory sexuality and stable and effective erectile function, the basic themes of the patient's overall quality of life remain intact.

Depression and anxiety often arise from the relationship with the outside world and from the daily confrontation with one's own otherness.

15.3.1 Sexological Notes

Even boys with multiple sclerosis (MS) can tell us much. In the study of Lew-Starowicz et al. [5]:

1. 52.9% showed erectile dysfunction.
2. 26.8% had a decrease in sexual desire.
3. 23.1% had difficulty in achieving orgasm.
4. 17.9% had difficulty in ejaculation.
5. Only 6% of patients had NOT discussed the problems of sexual function with their doctor and had not sought treatment for them.

From this it can be deduced that the study and analysis of the problems of patients with MS and, in general, of patients with neurological pathologies is not yet well developed.

Proposing a penile prosthesis implant for these patients, in particular, therefore means analyzing the patient's expectations, their sexual relationship, their anxiety and depression disorders, and their emotional, social, and relational difficulties with the outside world.

While a healthy sexuality may be a positive condition for the self-esteem and sexual role of these patients, it is not the solution to the emotional problems associated with neurological diseases.

A study in 1998 clearly showed the efficacy of penile prostheses with respect to intracavernous injection therapy. *Of the 65 patients in the study, only 41% were still using intracavernous therapy, while more than 70% of the patients were sexually active with the prosthesis.*

The most frequent reasons for discontinuing intracavernous therapy were *inadequate erections, lack of spontaneity in the sexual act, side effects, lack of a partner, and loss of sexual interest. In contrast, in the study there were only six discontinuations of implant use due to complications (infection, erosion, and malfunction) and seven for implant-independent reasons (lack of partner, loss of sexual interest, and comorbidity).*

15.4 Patients and Therapeutic Approaches

The variable is always and only the patient, above all, in young and older men who are coping every day with feelings of tiredness and bladder disorders; feelings of apathy alternating with dissatisfaction, otherness, and distrust; and fear of losing the partner or, worse, not being adequate (affectively and sexually).

The sexual history and the analysis of the moment of the neurological diagnosis seem to be the preliminary cornerstones for the preparation for a surgical implant of penile prostheses, in addition to:

1. Excluding psychiatric pathologies, dysmorphism.
2. Investigating the impact of the neurological pathology on the patient and on the family context.
3. Discovering with the patient, the body's areas of sensitivity and insensitivity.
4. The sex education received.
5. Investigating pornography or alcohol addiction or substance abuse.
6. Introduction of the use of vacuum device for preliminary andrological exercises half a month before the operation.
7. Analysis of expectations for improvement and/or deterioration of the patient's quality of life after penile prosthesis implantation.
8. Hypothesizing about the reactions of the partner to the use of the penile prosthesis.
9. Hypothesizing about the presence of the prosthesis with paid partners or with friends.
10. Implementation of a quality of life project that includes not only improved sexual function but also a more balanced desire and an attention to sexuality, in addition to improving mood stability, social interaction, and employability.
11. Constant follow-up to check with the patient the new life path.

Bioengineering has also gradually improved the technique of construction over time, and penile prostheses are now no longer a cause for mechanical failure and do not lead to postoperative complications such as infection or erosion, except in rare cases.

A 2015 study Yoon Seob et al. [6] showed that 42 patients (79.2%) out of 53 in total reported that the devices were easy to use, and 48 patients (90.6%) reported that the prostheses had adequate rigidity during intercourse. The overall satisfaction rate was 86.8%, and 43 patients pointed out that the implant improved their sexual life. A total of 44 patients (83%) would again undergo a penile implant, and 47 patients (88.7%) would advise a friend to undergo the same surgery. In contrast to the high rate of sexual satisfaction of the patient, only 32 patients (60.4%) responded that they had experienced an orgasm.

15.5 The Vacuum Device

The fact remains that the use of the vacuum device often inhibits the patient and the partner if they are not young. The recommendations and methods of use described by the psychosexologist should take into account the sensitivity and embarrassment of each member of the couple.

"*It is an andrological instrument aimed at a penile exercise, of the external covering and of the internal corps cavernosa...*" begins the psychosexologist, in response to the often hasty and technical explanation of the surgeon.

"But only he has to do it, right?" the partners often reply... "*don't I have to be there too while he is doing the vascularization excercise on his member?...don't we use it during sexual intercourse?...*"

Only after explaining to the partners that there is a similar gynecological instrument, especially after hysterectomy or vaginal plastic surgery, does the partners' initial sense of discomfort and reluctance diminish: "*Ah, I didn't know...but it will be different...in the design and in the way of using it. Who would have thought it, poor girls...*"

In a Catholic country such as Italy, it is often useful to shut out moral and ethical meaning from this practice which, initially, must be carried out every day.

Very often surgeons take it for granted that the vacuum should be accepted by the patient as "a form of exercise to improve penile extension and expansion." This could also be shared in a discussion between the patient and the surgeon.

The psychosexologist has no choice but to promote this practice to the couple, because often the patient needs to feel supported and understood by the partner, also in this "exercise."

Let us not forget that a couple with a neurological partner lives in a constant state of worry and concern about possible relapses and disease. *Thus, a prosthetic implant, if desired, and the use of vacuum device can be very invasive in the emotional nature of the couple.*

It is then a matter not of forcing the couple into a medicalized sexuality but of taking into account how they have experienced intimacy (in terms of quality, quantity, and frequency) in the years preceding the diagnosis and/or the prosthetic implantation, depending on the couple's age and on the history of the two.

All this helps the surgeon and the medical team not to underestimate the beliefs, values, and habits of the couple and, above all, to respect the idea of the sexuality of the patient and the partner. In fact, the continued practice with the vacuum device, if not supported by the partner, could soon become abandoned, casting the neurological patient and the partner into a constant anticipation of failure.

Keep in Mind

In such cases it is not necessary to number how many times the psychosexologist will repeat the methodology of vacuum device use because each time a doubt, a shyness, and a modesty of one or the other partner will emerge:

> *You know, we have never done strange things...we have always had a normal sex life...We are Catholics and these things make us uncomfortable...He won't always have to do these exercises, will he? Does he have to do his exercise in the same place?—Can he lock himself up in the bathroom?*

Until all these doubts are resolved by the psychosexologist, it is not possible to impose such a practice merely because it is prescribed by the rehabilitation protocol before and after surgery.

The patient must feel fully in tune with clinical practice, and if this is not possible, it is right to respect the sensitivity of the patient and partner. "*I'm sorry, I don't want to disappoint your commitment...may be we are not up to what you are offering us...*" could be the couple's first reaction.

No one can tell you how to live. Surgery requires rehabilitative practices that can be modified, depending on the sensitivity of the couple. Do not be afraid (psychosexologist)...*we will do it another way. We have learned new information together*"....

Leaving the patient to adapt, in terms of time and manner, to the surgical and rehabilitative phase is a method that strengthens therapeutic ties of trust and respect, without which surgery would have great margins of failure in meeting the needs of the patient and the couple.

On the perception of the validity of this surgical procedure

An innovative questionnaire—Quality of life and sexuality with penile prosthesis—exploring patient's perspectives on PP implantation, such as the impact on their quality of life, on their relationships, and on their self-esteem, has been recently validated, and this might represent a milestone in sexual medicine by improving the quality of evidence on PROs after PP implantation [7].

If in healthy patients the percentages, although striking, show some asymmetry, it is easy to deduce that the implantation of a penile prosthesis in a neurological patient shows many more variations: of satisfaction and disorientation, of rediscovered virility, and of loneliness.

The Case

Guido is a young man of 32 years. The neurologist who referred him has followed him since his diagnosis of multiple sclerosis. He has offered him psychotropic drugs for anxiety and depression, but Guido refused, preferring to meet a psychosexologist.

Guido's story appears complex. He studied at the conservatory: he is a conductor of orchestra, a graduate in piano and guitar, and a composer of film music.

But he is not working when I meet him. He appears anxious and with severe depressive behaviors and sexual and sleep disorders. He was 25 years old when he was struck by the first attack of multiple sclerosis: 2 months after the death of his mother from leukemia. At 28 and 30 years of age, the last attacks of the disease coincided with the end of his relationship with his long-time girlfriend (*She said she was not able to live with illness and well-being…*) and with the diagnosis of psoriasis of his younger brother, Davide.

15.6 Interview with Sexologist

"*It's a community of men my family*" explains Guido "*My older brother is a dentist, there is me, my brother Davide, an accountant and my father Silvio, a criminal lawyer. We all live in the same building. Each of us has a small apartment. All alone, except Davide who has been living with his partner for a year.*"

(Psychosexologist) "*What led you to turn to me? Why do you prefer therapy to a more practical pharmacological solution?*"

Guido replies that he is interested in overcoming the anxiety and depression that have plagued him since his mother's death, but he wants to talk about his "unexpressed virility."

He has had a penile prosthesis for a year and has not yet had sexual intercourse. "*I think I'm a plastic man*" says Guido "*I have several female friends, some know about my illness, but they treat me as if I were asexual…if greater intimacy arises… one way or another they move away…*"

Guido is not sure if he made the right choice when choosing a prosthetic implant "*The surgeon assured me that I would find myself again. I did some preliminary tests, and I understood I had not 'to be crazy' …and once home I was asked if I wanted to talk to someone…I asked myself 'talk about what? I have my neurologist'…*"

In fact, the neurologist was much more than a specialist for Guido: he was the doctor who visited the hospital even outside hours; he was the doctor who spoke to Guido's father if he seemed disappointed with their relationship. He had become "the navigator" of that community of men. But he was another man.

It was the neurologist who told him to talk to a therapist, a psychologist, and a sexologist.

(Psychosexologist): "*What do you hope to find through me*?"

Guido answers, crying "*I'm lost…all my family is lost after the loss of mum…My older brother started to use drugs in the evening; Davide is struggling with psoriasis all over his body…even on the genitals… and my father, for some time has been drinking…He denies it, but sometimes he can't stand up after dinner…he has missed court hearings, because he wasn't yet sober by the morning….*"

The patient appears to be looking for a female soul to cling to, because "*without a woman, our family has drifted…mother drove all of us, kept us together…but I, what can I offer a woman? How can she accept me as sick and with a 'fake penis?'… I was too hasty thinking that with a prosthesis, I would have solved the problem…*"

(Psychosexologist) "When was the last time you were all right sexually?"

"*4 years ago.*" Guido replies "*I was fine with Rossana (the long-standing girlfriend), with her the sex life was fine…I suffered from erectile dysfunction, and sometimes I couldn't ejaculate…She told me that everything was fine, that in time I would recover…and, when she had the possibility of a tour (…she was a cellist…), she didn't pass the possibility up and I didn't hear from her again…*"

Not by chance was Rossana "liked by my mother, because she told me 'she's patient and you are a right character'…but not so patient as to give me time to rebuild a future…maybe I got the prosthesis because I hoped for her return….If she had found me virile, maybe she would not have gone away…"

Everything had already been decided by doctors: diagnosis, therapy, surgery, and even the psychosexologist.

The same procedure could not be repeated "*I do not want to put myself on the list of those who, with much expertise, have guided you in your clinical choices. I propose to accompany you in time in a process of addressing your new project of being a man. But on an equal footing, together we will study the pros and cons of each situation, and you will choose the most realistic hypothesis for that moment.*"

Guido liked the idea and allowed me affectionately to call him "Maestro".

As an exception, the interviews were 20 in number and not 5–6 as usual, because Guido was alone and the interferon treatment had a significant effect on his physical stamina and mood.

After 6 months, Guido called me from Prague: he was recording a composition for a German film "*I'm with a 120-piece orchestra…I've been rehearsing for 8 hours…I'm very tired, but I feel like I'm in heaven…I wanted to tell you….You are the only one who can understand my effort and my joy…*"

Thanks to the interaction with the neurologist and Guido's father with whom I had two conversations, Guido managed to resume his interests and to convince his father to turn to Alcoholics Anonymous. It wasn't much work, but Guido continued to compose and to teach at the Conservatory, even when his hands no longer allowed him to play the piano and he switched to a computer keyboard.

> Sexuality began little by little with occasional encounters in between an orchestra rehearsal in Prague and a concert in Rome, a tour in Japan, and a rehearsal in Madrid. "*As you say, doctor* (Guido speaks), *I get tired of travelling, but it gives me the opportunity to do 'sexual exercise in the laboratory.' I meet nice partners, I don't fall in love, I spend one or more evenings with them, and I train my prosthesis...*"

The farewell was just as serene and consequential "*Now you no longer need me (the psychosexologist), so Maestro, it's time to say goodbye...*"

"*I don't know what to say* (Guido); *I know it's right...but if I would like to talk to you, will you be there?*"

> "(Psychosexologist) *If you have done your homework and have done everything to be happy, you won't need me. On days when you feel a little more human than usual .... you will remember what you learned for yourself. In moments of triumph, from orchestra to orchestra, it is right that this is celebrated alone ... In all these cases and when you are not thinking I will always be there ... In your memory ... and within you ...*"

15.7 Conclusions

Surgery in neurological patients requires a deep psychosexological approach, both preparatory to implantation and post-surgical. The partners, who are already largely overwhelmed by the physical symptoms and constant sensations of otherness and emotional fatigue, require for once to be considered "persons" and not only "complex neurological patients".

The sharing of their feelings and expectations about the outcome of prosthetic surgery is essential to avoid failures in the final satisfaction of the implant for the patient and the partner.

As is choosing, in terms of their religious, moral, ethical, and emotional beliefs, the least intrusive practices for rehabilitation and access to a sober and serene quality of life. Surgeons and psychosexologists can therefore be a coresponsive and flexible unit, as otherwise they can become for the patient and the partner an uncompromising team and an unwitting cause of emotional fatigue.

15.8 Self-Check Path

None of the questions below envisages a right and/or wrong answer. This is a way to learn from yourself and be more aware of your therapeutic style.

If a neurological patient comes to ask you to implant a penile prosthesis, do you make sure:

1. The motivation is deep, and you share it with the patient in clinical, relational, and emotional terms.
2. You ask for psychosexological counselling immediately.
3. That he has a fixed partner.
4. You review the patient's entire clinical history.
5. You see the request as the only solution to the erectile problem.
6. You try to explain the procedure to him.
7. You consider the possibility that the patient is not an eligible candidate for implantation.
8. You ask for further clinical investigations.
9. You listen at length to the patient's and the couple's motivation.
10. You ensure with the team that the patient and partner are in the best physical and emotional condition to cope with the prosthetic implant.

If the psychosexologist informs you that, in his/her opinion, the patient could suffer from psychosomatic, depressive, or anxiety disorders, do you:

1. Ask for a psychiatric counselling?
2. Postpone the implantation date to a time to be defined with the team?
3. Risk the patient's turning to another surgeon.
4. Ask the patient to attend a team meeting with the psychosexologist and other specialists on basic neurological pathologies?
5. Think that the psychosexologist is too fussy?
6. Review with the psychosexologist the patient's psychic, emotional and relational state, the couple's motivations, their religious beliefs, prejudices, and fears?
7. Agree more meetings with the patient so that the surgical and rehabilitation process is clear?
8. Ask the psychiatrist to prescribe antidepressant therapy to avoid postoperative psychic complications?

If a patient refuses to perform the exercises with the vacuum device, do you:

1. Inform him of the clinical consequences of such an omission?
2. Ask the psychosexologist for a deeper understanding of the patient's motivations and the social, religious, economic, and emotional basic ties that exist?
3. Leave it to the patient without objecting?
4. Review with the patient a range of more adaptive alternatives?
5. Ask for an interview in the presence of the partner to ask for support?
6. Agree with the psychosexologist on an individualized path so that the patient can make a conscious and serene decision?
7. Delegate the psychosexologist to find a solution?
8. Increase the number of checkups for the patient to review more often and reassess the situation?
9. Find it unbearable when patients don't understand the delicacy of your work?
10. Feel sure that every patient will offer you the means to find a rehabilitation strategy?

15.9 Medical History Questions

15.9.1 For the Patient

1. How did you arrive at this decision?
2. What kind of expectations do you have about the outcome of the prosthetic implant?
3. Do you think you have enough information from the surgeon? Do you want us to review the surgical procedure together?
4. What attempts have you made to improve sexuality before approaching a penile prosthesis implant?
5. Who knows of your decision?
6. What ideas and feelings come back during the day when you think about this surgery?
7. Who chose our center and how?
8. Did you feel welcomed by the medical and paramedical team?
9. In what spirit did you come here today? What do you expect from our meeting?
10. If you do not achieve the desired result, what do you think your future could be?

15.9.2 For the Partner

1. How do you see your partner right now?
2. Are you worried about him?
3. How do you see this surgical choice? Have you contributed to it or are you submitting to it?
4. Have you thus far been taken into account by the doctors and the paramedical team?

5. Who have you spoken to about this experience?
6. What do you think are the most difficult problems for your partner: hospitalization, anesthesia, surgery, the outcome of the surgery, your relationship as a couple?
7. For yourself, what do you fear the most?
8. How much has the neurological pathology of your partner affected your life, work, and social choices?
9. What do you hope will happen after the prosthetic operation?
10. Have you ever had any gynecological surgery?

15.9.3 For the Couple

1. Have the two of you had the opportunity to discuss your individual interviews with me?
2. Is there a particular thought that you focus on more often?
3. Has your motivation changed as you approach the possibility of dealing with the prosthetic operation?
4. How important is sexuality in your relationship?
5. What do you usually talk about, apart from neurological disease, symptoms, or therapies?
6. Outside the workplace, what kind of interests have you developed individually and together?
7. What could happen, either positive or less positive, in the relationship after the prosthetic implantation?
8. Do you have children? (If not: Have you ever wanted them? Which of you would most have hoped to become a parent?
9. Who currently is closest to you among your loved ones?
10. How do you overcome difficult moments? Do you talk about them?

References

1. Smith AE et al (2015) Sexual function, satisfaction and use of clinical procedures for sexual activity in middle-aged adults with long-term physical disabilities. Top Spinal Cord Inj Rehabil 21(3):227–232
2. Bombardier CH et al (2004) Symptoms of major depression in people with spinal cord injury: implications for screening. Arch Phys Med Rehabil 85(11):1749–1756
3. Khak M et al (2016) Evaluation of sexual function and its factors in men with spinal cord injury by using a questionnaire. Am J Mens Health 10(1):24–31
4. Cobo Cuenca AI et al (2015) Psychological impact and sexual dysfunction in men with and without spinal cord injury. J Sex Med 12(2):436–444
5. Lew Starowicz M et al (2014) Sexual dysfunction and sexual quality of life in men with multiple sclerosis. J Sex Med 11(5):1294–1301

6. Yoon Seob JI et al (2015) Long-term survival and patient satisfaction with inflatable penile prosthesis for the treatment of erectile dysfunction. Korean J Urol 56(6):461–465
7. Caraceni E et al (2014) A questionnaire for the evaluation of quality of life after penile prosthesis implant: Quality of life and Sexuality with Penile Prosthesis, (QolSPP). J Sex Med 11:1005–1012

Penectomy for Penile Malignancy Quality of Life and Sexual Disorders

16

Elena Vittoria Longhi and Leonardo Misuraca

16.1 Introduction

Squamous cell carcinoma (SCC) of the penis is a malignant disease, which accounts for 0.6% of all (malignant) neoplasms among men in the United States and Europe [1]. In 2012 the estimated number of new cases of penile cancer was 1570 with 310 deaths.

In the United Kingdom, it is estimated that some 350 patients are diagnosed with this pathology each year.

The incidence is 10% higher among men in developing countries in Asia, Africa, and South America. The most common age of onset is between 50 and 70 years [2].

Early diagnosis of the disease is of the utmost importance: andrological surgery can bring, depending on the case, a devastating, partial, or total disfigurement of the penis, with a survival rate of about 50% (>85% for patients with negative lymph nodes and 29–40% for patients with positive lymph nodes).

As the rarity of this pathology makes it difficult to perform prospective and randomized studies, it is of great importance that the patient is assisted with regard to emotional, relational, and quality of life issues, before and after surgery. A comprehensive understanding of how this disease impacts on social interactions, self-esteem, self-image, and quality of life can develop a complete and multidisciplinary approach:

Surgeon, Psychosexologist, Psychiatrist, and Nurses

This is also because the high rate of anxiety and the impossibility of obtaining long-term benefits from the results of surgery mean that these patients have to deal on a daily basis with the impossibility of loving, of making long-term plans, of resuming a satisfactory sexuality, of reestablishing a good relationship with their

E. V. Longhi et al., *Psychosexual Counseling in Andrological Surgery*,
https://doi.org/10.1007/978-3-319-99646-2_16

own body scheme, of dealing with everyday life without anxiety, and of counting on their partner and family.

Partial or total amputation of the penis in an adult person leads to depression, psychological disorders, and suicidal ideation.

16.2 The Scientific Literature

The risk of suicide among breast cancer patients was 37%, while among penile cancer patients, it could reach up to 50% [3].

A study by Maddineni et al. [4] evaluated 128 patients from six studies using 13 qualitative questionnaires to assess psychological well-being, quality of life, and sexual function.

The General Health Questionnaire (GHQ) showed that 40% of patients complained of a significant impairment of their quality of life, especially after undergoing severely mutilating surgical treatments.

The anxiety and depression score during hospitalization (HADS) showed up to 31% pathological anxiety in two studies.

One study used the DSM III R (*Diagnostic and Statistical Manual of Mental Disorders of Psychiatric Diseases*) with 53% evidence of mental pathology in patients with penile neoplasia and 40% evidence of social phobic, avoidance, and psychosis behaviors.

20–30% suffered from post-traumatic stress disorders.

The IIEF (the questionnaire that measures erectile function) showed in one study that as many as 67% of patients reported no sexual response, while 78% found pleasure neither in the sexual act nor with the new erection.

Using the FIFL-Meyer Life Satisfaction Checklist (Lisat 11), 50% of patients showed better sexual satisfaction [5], having undergone a less mutilating treatment with laser therapy.

Make a Note

1. Fourteen out of 18 patients reported a high frequency in erectile response.
2. While 3 out of 18 had not reached orgasm.
3. Six out of 18 had reduced sexual desire.
4. Twelve out of 18 had reduced sexual satisfaction compared to the presurgical period.

The study by Gulino et al. [6] compared the scores before the disease and after treatment and showed no significant differences.

Research by D'Ancona et al. [7] used the Global Sexual Behavior Questionnaire (QSFQ) and found that nearly 36% of patients treated with partial penectomy had no sexual function or had a moderately or severely reduced sexual function.

Finally, the study by Ficarra et al. [8] showed that patients had moderate sexual function scores in all surgical treatment groups, but patients with more mutilating surgery had lower scores.

From these studies, there emerges a picture of a negative impact on the well-being of patients, with psychiatric symptoms in up to 50% coupled with a feeling of unpleasantness toward their body, hatred and resentment toward life, and anger and depression at feeling victims of an illness they did NOT deserve.

16.3 The Andrological Aspects

Main recognized risk factors are an history of phimosis, chronic penile inflammation, balanitis xerotica obliterans, smoking, and HPV infection (especially HPV-16 and HPV-18). Furthermore, there is a frequent association with multiple sexual partners, unprotected intercourses, and low socioeconomic status.

Circumcision is an effective prophylactic measure, especially when performed in the neonatal period.

> In the majority of cases, penile cancer develops on the glans or prepuce as a flat or exophytic lesion, with or without a concomitant reddening or ulceration. Pain is uncommon as well as a foul odor. Diagnosis is basically clinic and starts from the physical examination which must include a careful palpation of both groins to evaluate inguinal lymph nodes. However, the most important diagnostic test is biopsy which should contain tissue beneath the visible lesion in order to stage the disease.

No specific laboratory studies or tumor markers have a diagnostic role in penile cancer.

Finally, ultrasound, MRI, CT, and PET scan are useful for local and distance disease spread evaluation. They allow a complete staging which is primary for a careful treatment planning.

Therapeutic options depend on the histology, location and size of the lesion, and the presence or not of palpable inguinal nodes.

For superficial lesions, topical treatment with 5-fluorouracil or imiquimod, or alternatively laser ablation, can be a minimally invasive treatment with minimum psychological impact.

In selected patients, basically young men with small (<3 cm) noninvasive cancers, radiotherapy is a valid alternative to surgery with the potential to maintain potency. Unfortunately, the necessity of a high dose may produce urethral strictures, fistulae, or penile necrosis with pain and edema.

Frozen sections at the time of surgery are often helpful in determining the resection adequacy. When the tumor involves the glans and distal shaft, a glandulectomy or partial amputation is appropriate, and a 2 cm margin is necessary. Local wedge

Nevertheless, surgery remains the most common treatment for all stages of penile cancer. Early diagnosis generally allows an organ-sparing surgery. In fact, superficial lesions can be treated with circumcision if tumor is confined to the prepuce, local excision, or Mohs micrographic surgery. It implicates removing a layer of the skin that the tumor may have invaded and then checks the sample under a microscope right away. If it contains cancer, another layer is removed and examined. This process is repeated until the skin samples are found to be free of cancer cells.

resection is also another option, but it is associated with a recurrence rate of 50%. If wedge resection or partial penectomy does not provide an adequate margin, a total penectomy should be considered, and if the amount of residual penis and urethra is inadequate to allow micturition while standing, perineal urethrostomy can be performed. Urination can still be controlled because the urethral sphincter is spared, but the patient will have to sit down to urinate, changing his social habits.

When inguinal nodes are palpable or abnormal at CT scan or MRI, a bilateral lymphadenectomy should be performed, even if this is still an area of debate and no clear recommendations can be given.

Basically, it is performed several weeks following partial or total penectomy and after a short course of antibiotic therapy.

Imaging studies and sentinel node biopsy can be helpful in identifying patients with micrometastatic disease who can benefit from lymphadenectomy.

Finally, chemotherapy is an option for patient with systemic disease and limited metastatic load. It can be performed in adjuvant or neoadjuvant setting followed by radical surgery in patients with non-resectable or recurrent lymph node metastases.

Because tumors can recur locally or distally, long-term observation is necessary. Follow-up timing depends on disease characteristics and therapy performed.

16.4 The Notable Absentees

- No statistical survey, however, reports the feeling of the partner, the sense of repulsion toward the patient's body, and the loss in the face of changes in his mood and at the end of each partnership project.
- In addition, they often suffer estrangement from friends, relatives, and even children.

16.5 Partner's Feelings 1

"*I feel lost, restless and alone*" reveals Marianna 49, partner of a patient with penile cancer "*At the time of diagnosis I thought only about the choice of the best surgeon and the most specialized facility to be sure that Alberto (the patient, 52 years) was in good hands. I felt sorry for him for what had happened to him, and I admired him greatly for the perseverance with which he had surgery. But the amputation of the penis was a real tragedy for our family…My children say…'Mum, it isn't him anymore, leave…don't you see how strange he is?' He's always intolerant, in a bad mood and keeps taking sick days from work…he spends whole days in bed…and when he approaches me…I'm ashamed to say I feel disgust…My mother-in-law doesn't want us to go to her place for lunch on Sundays because she says she is afraid of Alberto's reactions…the other Sunday he broke a dish because his mother hadn't cooked him what he wanted….He doesn't wash himself, he doesn't shave for days…When I go to work, I'm always afraid that I'm suddenly going to get a call because Alberto has done something…He doesn't want to see friends… and the other day, he had an accident…he suddenly crashed into a motorcyclist…My children avoid him…especially Clara, the little one, because she cries every time Alberto gets irritated about something. Luca, my eldest son, worries me… 'if he dares to touch you' he told me one evening 'I'll nail him to the wall'…The tension in the house is always very high, and I don't know what to do…I can't accept that my life has ended at 49….*"

16.6 Partner's Feelings 2

"*I work with my father in an architectural studio*" *says Pietro, 28.* "*From the time he underwent partial surgical treatment for penile cancer, I had to protect myself from him…It's not bad I know…but depression is eating him up and one day he asked me 'Would you die with me?' I was dumbstruck for a few moments and then 'Don't you think about your mother and me?' And he says 'it's over for me'…He comes to the studio, falls asleep, forgets to call suppliers and appointments with customers…and if I say to him 'stay at home, don't worry'…he looks at me badly and says 'What are you saying?' My mother cries with me, she cries with her friends, she cries with my grandmother… She's in pieces…My sister is eight months pregnant and we hear her on the phone…Mum is afraid for my sister's unborn child and health…I asked my mother to sell the studio…I still don't know what to do, but my father at this moment is unhealthy for everyone…*"

16.7 Even Conservative Surgery Has Its Pros and Cons

A recent study by Kyle Scarberry in [9] reported a survey of six patients who had received penile cancer surgery at the Cleveland Clinic between 2003 and 2012. The quality of erectile and urinary function was evaluated.

1. Three patients reported having normal erections but described unpleasant intercourse.
2. The other three patients reported no sexual activity and denied sexual desire.
3. All patients reported mild urinary symptoms, including 18% flow decrease and 67% incomplete bladder emptying sensation.
4. Eighty-three percent of patients report that urinary symptoms did not interfere with their daily lives.

However, surgeons are only concerned with information about symptoms, urinary and sexual practice, NOT one's own identity, and "the fact that you find yourself being something that you are afraid even to identify. Certainly I'm not the man I was before" confirms Paolo, 56 "But who wants to listen to you? Who wants to listen to a hybrid, an anomaly of nature, and a waste of humanity? Who can such a creature be of use to? Why should my wife and children love me?

Kieffer et al. [10] evaluated the impact of primary partial surgery, penectomy (penile amputation), and lymphadenectomy on the sexuality and quality of life of patients.

The 147 patients recruited between 2003 and 2008 were given questionnaires: IIEF-15, SF-36, IOC version 2, and some questions about urinary function.

Only 90 patients answered the questionnaires.

Make a Note

1. Patients undergoing partial penectomy reported more problems than those treated with penectomy, especially regarding the aesthetic appearance and the lack of orgasm.
2. Men who underwent lymphadenectomy reported more disorders in the management of daily life and urinary function.

This is where the scientific literature ends, but clinical practice teaches us more. There is no doubt that this disease requires the patient to be cared for from the moment of diagnosis.

The psychosexologist, in particular, will alternate between individual interviews with the patient, interviews with the couple, and individual interviews with the partner.

16.8 From Taking on the Patient to Post-surgical Rehabilitation

16.8.1 With the Patient

Keep in Mind 1
Preliminary interviews for surgery will include:

1. Biographical and clinical history of the patient.
2. The impact of the diagnosis.
3. The anticipatory sensations of castration, loss of sexual role, and change in body scheme.
4. Preliminary study of the body map and of the physical-emotional sensations of the patient in his current state.
5. The in-progress hypothesis of how sensations could change shortly before entering the operating theatere.

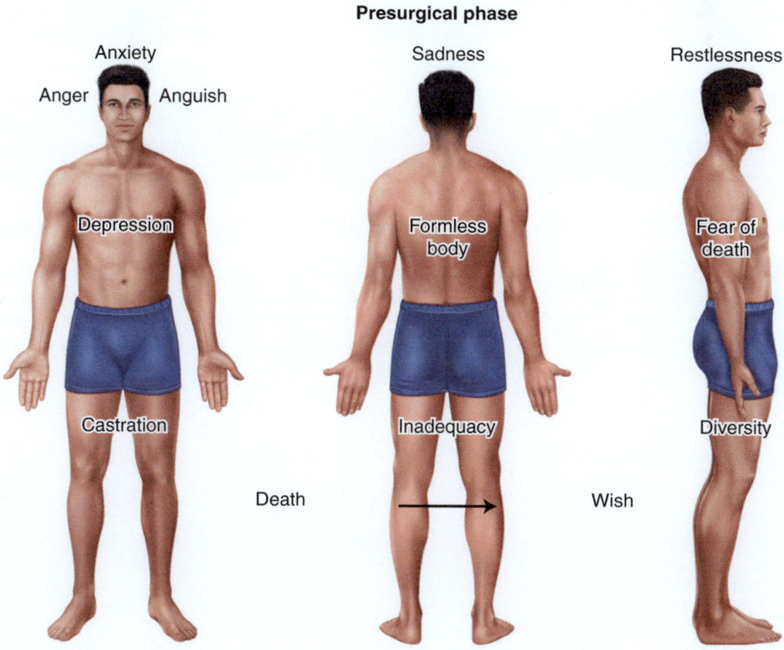

Keep in Mind 2

Interviews concerning hospitalization (Fig. B):

1. The variation of emotions and body sensations following post-traumatic stress from surgery
2. The de-responsibilization of the patient from distressing or panic sensations, consequent to post-surgical stress and NOT consequent to the inadequacy of the patient.
3. Nursing care and observation of the surgical outcome
4. The function of the nurse in self-learning regarding the medication
5. Interaction with the nurse in the first sensations of annoyance, discomfort, pain, and disorientation
6. The usefulness of body maps built with the psychosexologist in the presurgical phase and which described the emotional and symptomatic path

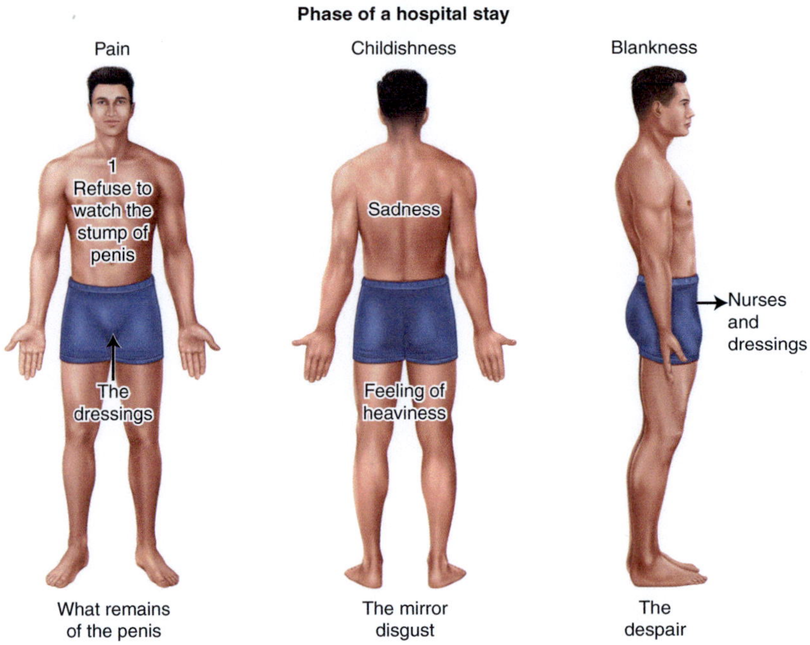

Keep in Mind 3

Interviews concerning rehabilitation (Fig. C):

1. Post-traumatic stress as a restructuring period of virility
2. The new self-esteem
3. From disorientation to a new human project in terms of HEALTH, AESTHETIC, and PLEASURE
4. The virtuous sensations (will to succeed, to resume the virile role in the family and at work) and the vicious (loss, depression, apathy, desire to let go … desire to die)
5. The new motivations of life. People who love me and who believe in me

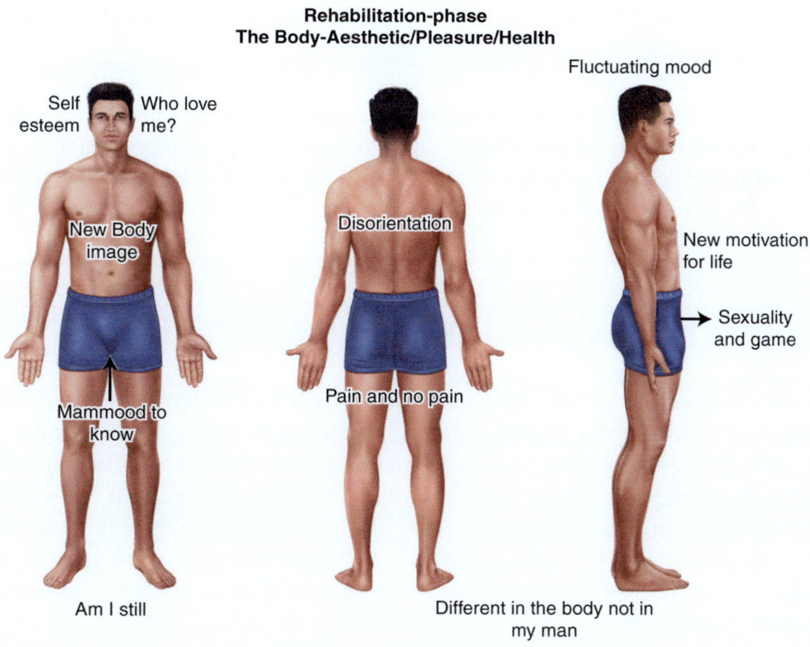

16.9 Recurrence

Most penile cancer recurrences develop within 5 years of primary treatment. Studies have shown that within 2 years of surgery following the first diagnosis, 66%, 86%, and 100%, respectively, of local, regional, and distant recurrences occur. Early diagnosis requires frequent follow-ups and constant self-examination by patients through self-palpation.

Most local recurrences can be successfully controlled without endangering long-term survival, often with penis-saving surgical techniques. The rate of recurrence in these patients varies between 20 and 50%.

Regional recurrence rates in pN0 patients are 0–10%, while in pN+ patients, the recurrence rate is 20–45%. These percentages depend on the stage, degree, and state of HPV and the presence of lymphovascular invasion.

Most distant recurrences are incurable as they are invariably accompanied by an advanced disorder. Patients with recurrences beyond the groin are candidates for palliative treatment or inclusion in clinical trials.

During the first 2 years, a 3-monthly follow-up is recommended in patients who have undergone penile retention techniques and 6-month intervals for patients undergoing penile amputation. Follow-up of regional lymph nodes consists of ultrasound with fine needle aspiration cytology (FNAC) as well as an objective examination for the presence of a palpable disease. The role of self-examination by the patient also should be repeatedly recommended.

16.10 The Therapeutic Relationship with the Nurses

The development of collaboration between nurses and patients with penile cancer aims to increase the patient's decision-making power in the treatment process. Effective communication creates and maintains a good relationship; this is essential but little considered, and this affects the degree of patient involvement. The reciprocity of intentions and the negotiation of the objectives to be achieved allow the provision of focused and shared care services. A prerequisite for a therapeutic relationship between the nurse and the patient is a deep understanding of the patient.

- *The psychosexologist in this sense can be a "facilitator" in the process of communication with the patient, the surgeon, and the nursing team.*
- The nurse is the professional figure who spends the most time in contact with the patient and therefore has a considerable opportunity to influence the patient's behavior and attitudes [11]. *The relationship that is established is a vehicle for the patient to develop confidence, comfort, respect, and involvement in the management of the disease* [11].

The traditional view of the patient's position in the treatment process is changed, having been replaced by the expectation that the patient will be an active and involved subject [12, 13], provided that the nurse's attitudes, strategies, and skills favor his participation, motivation, degree of satisfaction with the treatment, and the reduction of the level of stress and anxiety [12, 13].

Let us think, for example, of the administration of treatment accompanied by further encouragement of the nurse to use the dispensing of drugs as a moment of relationship, of sharing…"*You look better today…These are the prescribed treatments, and I am sure that your will to get better will have more than the desired effect…*"

Patient participation is defined as a dynamic process that changes over time [13] and that takes place with the individual as the central element. Participation is linked to the patient's involvement in the decision-making process regarding possible therapeutic alternatives and implies the presence of terms associated with it such as equality, negotiation, and responsibility [13].

The concept of equality leads to that of preserving the human dignity of the patient; this issue is addressed daily in nursing practice and can be understood as a component of preserving health [14]. The patient-centered care process is a solution to the de-humanizing aspects of hospitalization [15].

Who is coming to visit you today?…I'm sure you will be happier tonight… You're lucky…there are always lots of people at visiting time for you…don't get tired…"

- Preserving and conserving the dignity of the patient within the care relationship is considered one of the most important ethical aspects of caring [14], *even if only when the patient and nurse are complicit in observing the outcome of surgical treatment for the first time with the aid of a mirror.*
- With whom else could the patient share the fear, the disgust, and the feeling of discomfort of a disfigured pelvic part, with bruises, wounds, and swelling?
- With whom else could he share those anxious and fearful silences?
- Who, better than the nurse, could share the emotion and tears of such a harsh trial? *This too is part of the therapeutic process of treatment and rehabilitation.*

16.11 Conclusions

Penile cancer is undoubtedly a malignant pathology that consumes to the maximum the emotional, psychological, and relational resources of the patient and the family, as well as those of the therapeutic team. In these cases, the caregivers and doctors not only invest their professionalism; they must go further, considering also their human investment, without ever losing the sense of their role and their therapeutic responsibility. Surgeons, doctors, nurses, and psychosexologists must engage in a team investment that is proportional to the feelings of the patient and his family members while respecting their own limitations, which are determined by the disease and sometimes by its progression, despite the clinical efforts invested.

In this as in no other pathology, post-surgical rehabilitation is a consequence of the prolonged interest of the therapeutic team in the daily life of the patient.

Case Illustration

The voices and revelations of patients

The Feel of the Patient 1

When I learned from Dr…that She was a woman, I thanked heaven. I would never have had the courage to speak to a man. What could he have found 'healthy' faced with me? Even if he had understood me, I would have thought that he was a hypocrite…like those who say to me 'I'm so sorry…you'll make it, you'll see.' Great prospect. I already feel like a lifeless larva, and when they castrate me…how could it be better?…I'm sorry for my wife. She is my second wife. She's younger, she's 15 years younger than me…I have already told her that after the surgery, we'll go to a lawyer and we'll separate…I can't tie her to me…I'm a hybrid of a man and I don't want to bother with others anymore….

The Feel of the Patient 2

(61-year-old patient) Sometimes I look at the surgeon, and it seems to me that he doesn't tell me the whole truth. Besides 'cutting me into pieces, what can he do?' I trust him, but he too depends, like me, on the surgical outcome and on good luck. I've never been lucky, and maybe this is the right time to take leave of the world… .I lost my father when I was 8 years old. My older sister was in an institution in her teens because our grandmother said she was crazy. My mother committed suicide when she knew she had an incurable disease…and me, what should I do?…Every time I try to share these things with doctors they look frightened and they change the subject…Why is it that you (a psychosexologist) are different? I'd pay a pretty penny to know…

The Feel of the Patient 3

(Patient 50 years) When as a child my mother told me 'you're too hypersensitive' I thought for years that it was an illness. If a friend treated me badly, I would say to myself 'calm down, you're sick, you're hypersensitive…' Now I'd like my mother to be here to deal with this real disease…I became what she (the mother) had always wanted: an engineer, like my father. I got married and my wife betrayed me… because of my hypersensitivity I chose to leave the home...I felt bad around those who had trampled on my affections. I would like to do it...Doctor (psychosexologist)...I would like to be able to live for a while...I do not want to die. My new partner tells me that I have 'nine lives like cats,' but I would like to spend what I have left serene. Will I be a castrated man? I will understand what it means to be castrated...I'm so afraid, I cry every night, and...I don't blame myself...I take my mother's last letter to bed...I know it by heart...but it makes me feel less alone...Will you (psychosexologist) be there during my stay?...

The Feel of the Patient 4

(55 years old patient)...I've never talked so freely about myself...My friends call me 'mummy' because I listen to everyone and nobody ever knows too much about me... What can I tell you? I have a small window fitting company: I install windows of all kinds. I built it up on my own...My mother would have liked a scholarly son or a priest...I didn't even think about it... I got married, I had three children and two work with me. Marta the girl is a nurse...She's the one who looks after me and gives me courage...but I know how much she suffers...I hope to have time to make a will and leave the company to my children...I can't leave them with so many problems...If it were left to me, I wouldn't even have the surgery....My daughter insists so much and I don't want to leave her with a sense of guilt...Now I sound like an angel, but that's not the case...A few days ago I shouted at her (the daughter) 'Do you want a castrated father at all costs? Is this your love?'...I haven't slept all night...I'm afraid Dr., I disgust myself...I look in the mirror now and say to myself 'look, you look like you've got mange...' And then it will be worse...I've already thought that I won't look at my penis anymore...If I live...they can send a nurse to my home...to medicate me, wash me...and talk a little...as long as I can...

16.12 Conclusions

Penile cancer is an uncommon but psychologically devastating condition. A mix of embarrassment, fear, and personal neglect leads patients to a delayed diagnosis which worsens the prognosis and the likelihood of survival, forcing surgeons to opt for partial or total penile amputation. These represent a more invasive surgical approach with huge impact on social habits and severe repercussions on sexual life and coupledom.

16.13 Self-Check Path

As always, there are no right or wrong answers. This is just a way to learn for oneself, discover one's limits, and improve one's therapeutic style.

1. Faced with a relapse, is it easier for you to feel a sense of helplessness, anger, or inadequacy in your clinical knowledge?
2. Does dealing with a disabling surgical treatment make you think: "I have to do it to save the patient's life," "I wish he had turned to another surgeon," "it's an interesting case to write an article about," etc. ?
3. For you, are the patient's partner and family members an additional reason for responsibility and discomfort, a support team with the help of the psychosexologist, or a further problem?
4. In your therapeutic team, could the figure of the psychosexologist, the figures of nurses who are too dedicated, and the figures of volunteers who cause confusion in the department be superfluous?

5. When you face a patient to whom you have to communicate a diagnosis of malignant penile cancer, do you put it in the most professional and scientific way, avoid the patient's asking too many questions and communicate the surgical procedure, or reassure him that you will do everything so that the treatment is not too harmful?
6. During hospitalization, would you like the patient to have no post-surgical complications, bear the pain, not complain too much, or not report self-destructive ideas?
7. Psychiatric counselling is in these cases a routine visit for the patient, counselling to be asked for only in serious cases, or one of the counselling services provided by the multidisciplinary therapeutic team?
8. If the patient were separated or a widower, would you feel you had to supervise him with closer follow-ups, would you involve the social services, or would you start him on a joint therapy with psychosexologist and psychiatrist?

16.14 Medical History Questions

16.14.1 For the Patient

1. What did you think when the surgeon told you your diagnosis?
2. What are the feelings or thoughts you most often reflect on?
3. Who knows about your diagnosis?
4. Do you ever have the feeling that this is just a bad nightmare and not a malignant diagnosis?
5. What projects did you have to set aside on the occurrence of the diagnosis?
6. What frightens you most about the surgery?
7. Is the fact that you will be followed even after your surgery and your return home a situation that lifts you or worries you?
8. Are you worried about your wife? Do you think you have the necessary strength to overcome this situation?
9. What do you fear most about the change in your body scheme?

16.14.2 For the Partner

1. What is it that worries you most about your husband's reactions at the moment?
2. You look worried, what disturbs you the most? That your husband can't overcome the trauma or that he doesn't feel ready for all this?
3. Who is close to you at the moment?
4. Have you talked to each other (the partner and the patient) about the situation?
5. How did your children react?
6. What do they know in the workplace about this situation? Has he asked for time off?
7. Have you thought how your life might be after the surgery?
8. What do you most want to happen?

16.14.3 For the Couple

1. What significance have you given to the discussions with the psychosexologist so far?
2. How do you plan to overcome the moments of greatest fragility of one or the other partner? How have you done this in other situations?
3. Who, in your experience, is more tenacious in difficult situations?
4. What projects would you not like to give up after your discharge from hospital?
5. How important has sexuality been to your relationship so far?
6. What do you fear will happen in your life as a couple if your surgical treatment prevents you from having a satisfactory sexuality?
7. How do you think the rapport with your partner's body will be?

References

1. Pettaway CA et al (2007) Penile cancer. In: Wein AJ et al (eds) Campbell-Walsh urology, vol 207, 9th edn. Saunders, Philadelphia, pp 959–992
2. Pow Sang MR et al (2010) Epidemiology and history of penile cancer. Urology 76:S2–S6
3. Camidge DR et al (2007) Hospital admissions and deaths about self-inflicted wounds and accidents within 5 years from the international cancer diagnosis: a national study in Scotland, United Kingdom. Br J Cancer 96:752–757
4. Maddineni SB et al (2009) Identifying the needs of patients with cancer of the penis: a systemic review of the quality of life, psychosexual and psychosocial literature on penile cancer. BMC Urol 9:8–18
5. Romero FR et al (2005) Sexual function after partial penectomy for penile cancer. J Urol 66:1292–1295
6. Gulino G et al (2007) Distal urethral reconstruction of the Glans penis cancer: results of a new technique to 1 year of follow-up. J Urol 178:941–944
7. D'Ancona CA et al (1997) Quality of life after partial penectomy for penile cancer. J Urol 50:593–596
8. Ficarra V et al (2000) General health and psychological well-being in patients undergoing surgery for Urologic malignancies. Urol Int 65:130–134
9. Scarberry K et al (2015) Results for organ sparing surgery for cancer of the penis. Sex Med 3(2):62–66
10. Kieffer JM et al (2014) Quality of life for patients treated for penile cancer. J Urol 192(4):1105–1110
11. Ku TK, Minas H (2010) *Development of the nursing relationships scale: a measure of interpersonal approaches in nursing care*. Int J Ment Health Syst 4:12
12. Sahlsten MJ, Larsson IE, Sjöström B et al (2007) *Patient participation in nursing care: towards a concept clarification from a nurse perspective*. J Clin Nurs 16(4):630–637
13. Sahlsten MJ, Larsson IE, Sjöström B et al (2008) *An analysis of the concept of patient participation*. Nurs Forum 43(1):2–11
14. Anderberg P, Lepp M, Berglund AL et al (2007) *Preserving dignity in caring for older adults: a concept analysis*. J Adv Nurs 59(6):635–643
15. Hobbs JL (2009) *A dimensional analysis of patient-centered care*. Nurs Res 58(1):52–62

Orchiectomy for Testicular Malignancy Sexual Disorders and Quality of Life

17

Elena Vittoria Longhi and Giorgio Franco

17.1 Introduction

Solid testicular cancer is the most common neoplasm in males of adult and adolescent age, between 15 and 29 years. It represents 21.4% of cancers in this age group, which contrasts with 2% of the testicular cancer prevalence among children aged 1–14 years and 7% among adults aged 30–45 years [1].

Survival rates at 5 years after diagnosis range from 71 to 99%, depending on the extent of the metastases of the disease. Young patients therefore live a significant part of their lives as "survivors" of testicular cancer, and their physical, emotional, and sexual vulnerability should not be underestimated; on the contrary, everyday life and quality of life are always much constrained.

Although the scientific literature has devoted little attention to the diagnosis of testicular cancer in young people under 15 years of age and the frequency of this disease is 2.7 times greater in individuals aged between 15 and 29 years, it has in fact increased rapidly among very young children [2].

17.2 Diagnosis and Treatment

Diagnosis is usually made by physical examination or self-palpation by the patient with the finding of an abnormal testicular mass or nodule, followed by scrotal ultrasound confirmation. Sometimes scrotal pain is the first symptom; in other instances an incidental diagnosis is made during the workup for infertility, which includes a scrotal ultrasound.

Tumor markers (AFP, BHCG, LDH, PLAP) are usually performed, but their negativity does not rule out the presence of the tumor. Additional investigations, usually performed after surgery, include chest-abdomen CT scan or MRI or PET/CT scan.

Surgical treatment of choice is inguinal orchiectomy. However, in selected cases (small nodules, bilateral tumors, patients with single testis), an organ-sparing approach

E. V. Longhi et al., *Psychosexual Counseling in Andrological Surgery*,
https://doi.org/10.1007/978-3-319-99646-2_17

such as testicular tumorectomy can be adopted. In patients with suspected secondary lymph node disease, a retroperitoneal lymphadenectomy might be indicated.

Radical inguinal orchiectomy is the definitive procedure to permit histology evaluation of the primary tumor and to provide local tumor control. It consists of a 3–5 cm inguinal incision with clamping and section of cord and delivery of the testis through the incision. Cord isolation used to be performed inside the inguinal channel with the section of cord at the internal inguinal ring. Nowadays minimal skin incision and simple section of the cord at the external inguinal ring are commonly accepted. Therefore, the invasiveness of this surgery has been greatly reduced, while the patient compliance has accordingly increased.

A testicular prosthesis is usually allocated in the scrotum at the end of the procedure in order to minimize the patient's psychological burden secondary to the postoperative aesthetic impairment.

Semen cryopreservation is indicated in some patients, particularly in those who should undergo adjuvant chemo- or radiotherapy or retroperitoneal lymphadenectomy.

Although studies have shown that cryopreserved sperm is subsequently rarely used for fertility purposes in these patients, the psychological advantage of having stored sperm is well known.

17.3 Sex and the Heart: What Do Scientific Studies Suggest?

That being said, testicular cancer involves a male organ which is highly associated with the perception of virility, body identity, sexual function, fertility, and the relationship with women.

Melissa Y Carpenter PhD et al. [3] reviewed the scientific literature to see if the relationships between couples, the affectivity of single patients, and the physical and emotional development of subjects with testicular cancer had ever been investigated. Only three studies had approached these issues, interviewing patients who had survived testicular neoplasm with an average age of 32–35 years [4, 5]

17.3.1 What Was Revealed?

Patients who survived the neoplastic pathology and who, at the time of diagnosis, were engaged in a long-term affective relationship describe a further physical and emotional improvement after surgical treatment, due to the greater affective and empathic closeness of the partner, and also report greater social support, revaluation of self-esteem, and better humor compared to patients who, from the time of diagnosis and throughout subsequent treatment, did not have relatives and friends at their side [6].

Keep in Mind

A percentage of these patients, on the other hand, report a worsening of conflict within the couple and of friendship and/or social relations, until they reach a real closure. For this portion of patients, the diagnosis and treatment of cancer lead to a greater feeling of self-destructiveness.

Fifty-two percent of survivors with relational difficulties and 55.9% of spouses of survivors indicate, after diagnosis and treatment, further financial worries and fear of talking about neoplasm, the possibility of recidivism, the implications for the future, and of the impossibility of seeing oneself in a peaceful old age.

These problems were aggravated, according to the interviewees, by the impossibility of talking about them with their spouse, who was already overwhelmed by anxiety and concern about the diagnosis and the prospect of an uncertain future.

Hence, certain drastic choices regarding the "ending of relationships" could be caused, not only by a poor understanding of each other's feelings but also by poor or no communication within the couple. This is then extended to friends or acquaintances [7].

Take-Home Message

Furthermore, being single at the time of diagnosis seems to provide an additional vulnerability that persists even when survivors develop a partner relationship after the completion of post-diagnosis treatment.

"...you are always a cancer patient"...begins Claudio, 37 "whatever you say or do, especially after getting married, you are blamed ...as an act of selfishness...' the family you wanted for yourself!...you had to marry a carer... wives need serenity, not problems' and you feel good for nothing...to the point that I wonder if it wouldn't have been better to let go and do nothing after the diagnosis...."."

In addition, other patients, commenting on the worsening quality of life, report such, especially in the sexual sphere, lamenting erectile dysfunction and poor orgasmic satisfaction, despite higher levels (mentally at least) of sexual desire [8].

In contrast to Brodsky's study, other research has found few problems with impotence, decreased desire, sexual dissatisfaction, sexual frequency, or lack of communication between partners regarding intimacy.

Among survivors aged over 40 years, research on sexual function before and after treatment for testicular cancer found a moderate degree of sexual dysfunction, low frequency of intercourse, and insufficient orgasmic satisfaction [9–11].

17.4 Mood Disorders

In these patients there was a greater presence of an anxiety syndrome, especially after treatment, poor libido, and a lack of self-confidence regarding sexual function, to the detriment of orgasmic pleasure, so much so that sexual inhibition of the central nervous system during periods of high stress is hypothesized [12].

In all patients surviving a diagnosis and treatment of testicular neoplasm, anxiety and depression syndromes would be present from 10 to 20% and may be associated with altered levels of gonadotropins. Just as patients who underwent retroperitoneal lymph node dissection (RPLND) or secondary resection after chemotherapy reported severe sexual efficiency problems, compared to patients treated with chemotherapy alone [13].

Finally, other research involving follow-ups long after diagnosis and treatment for testicular neoplasm (about 5–10 years) reported that sexual problems seem to split along age lines, with major ejaculatory dysfunctions among those between 20 and 39 years and erectile and desire disorders among those between 40 and 59 years. Dysfunctions are already present in 40% of patients 2 years after treatment.

The causes? Lack of a complicit partner, lower than normal testosterone rates, associated radiotherapy and chemotherapy treatments [6, 11].

In the end, however, all patients vaguely reported a lack of information regarding sexuality or postponed the discussion with specialists on this issue before and after the various clinical treatments.

Case Illustration 1

His Voice

"...at the time of diagnosis I had a girlfriend," Sergio, 37 "Monica (the girlfriend) seemed ready to face the diagnosis and the surgery with me...in fact it was she who chose the best surgeon, the best Health Facility, she who encouraged my parents... Then, in fact, the day they operated on me...there was my older brother with me...He was the one who played a 'father' to me...He encouraged me, he told me 'you did well, you evicted the squatter (the tumor)'...He took days off work and was with me every day of my stay...He brought me Monica's greetings, he told me that Monica was not well...I even worried...Then, by text message, she left me "I'm sorry. We've known each other for three months but I can't stay close. I love you...."

Case Illustration 2

Her Voice

"I met Edoardo, just while he was in hospital" Valeria 35 "My brother was his roommate I thought he was a nice guy, he never complained...he made witty jokes and talked about football with my brother. He was discharged before Franco (the brother) and one day he came to see him. 'What a nice thought.' I thought. Maybe out of gratitude I accepted his first invitation...Now I find myself once again in the hospital with him (Edoardo)...we have problems, we quarrel about everything...I love him but I don't want to spend my whole life always in the hospital...I have already lost my father, two years ago...With my brother it has gone well so far...I don't know what to do...Sexuality is also a disaster...I don't feel great excitement..."

17.5 Information on Tomorrow's Sexuality

This is the dominant point. Although the synergy between andrologists and psycho-sexologists has improved, the scheduling of interventions on these issues, in order to prepare patients and partners in advance, at whatever age, for changes in sexual life and body perception, is not always agreed.

The surgical experience is largely correct when it states, "the patient, faced with a diagnosis of testicular cancer, only thinks of saving his life. He doesn't care about sexuality..."

Take-Home Message

On the other hand, post-traumatic stress for the patient begins at the time of diagnosis and *not* after treatment for testicular neoplasm. A sympathetic and parasympathetic system prevents him from having an objective perception of reality. Anguish and fear disrupt awareness, and fear of death prevails [14].

Patients also talk to surgeons and adapt to their approach and language.

The psychosexologist, if present at the time of diagnosis, is a reassuring figure, seemingly saying to the patient "I will monitor your emotional and mental ups and downs, but I assure you that you will not be alone when you face the new life of the survivor ..."

Clinical experience over the years has taught me not to be invasive and, if anything, to look the patient and partner in the eyes, smiling, showing silent and complicit empathy.

The moment of the patient's disorientation was captured only at the end of the pivotal conversation with the surgeon, "well then doctor, are you going to operate? ..." or "chemotherapy and radiotherapy ... what do I do about my job? Am I going to be ill...?," with a complicit look to the surgeon, I say *"If you have a moment of patience we can talk about how to deal with everything...before and after the treatment..."*

Looks, smiles, a relaxed face, and maintaining a distance not too close nor too far from the surgeon and halfway between patient and andrologist. Nonverbal communication is very important in these cases because it implies that the staff are calm, they know what to do and how to do it, and above all they have thought about "from pre- through posttreatment" according to whether the patient is very young, a young adult, or an adult, with a partner, single, or homosexual.

Case Illustration 3

His Voice

> *"Anna is a woman with a strong character" Guido, 40 "She never gives up... always keeps on top of everything...When we learned the diagnosis she told me 'we will be like two peas in a pod'...we went through all the treatment and at every cycle of chemotherapy she looked worried, she couldn't bear to see me*

feeling sick and sometimes, bluntly, she said to me 'think that you are telling that tumor to piss off' ... She lost a lot of weight ... I feel guilty when I see her so messed up ... I say, 'get better' ... and she says 'are you saying that you don't like me anymore?'...it's not like that...but neither of us thinks about sexuality. I'm afraid...I still haven't overcome all the suffering of the treatment...I feel like a different man than before. Then ... there is always the fear of a relapse and the thought of leaving Anna alone ..."

Case Illustration 4
Her Voice

"I don't deny it: I'm so afraid of losing him" says Alexis 39 years old "And this thought is with me every day. After the orchidectomy the surgeon reassured us that Marco (her husband) was out of danger ... A year after the surgery the fear remains and at every check-up I feel I can't do it ... Marco would like a son but I'm afraid of being widowed with a small child ....The surgeon had not told me that I would be carrying the burden of the disease on my shoulders forever ... That's why I asked to talk to you Doctor ... (psychosexologist) Everyone has done a lot for Marco ... and it's right, for goodness' sake ... They have looked after him well ... but me? Who has ever asked me simply, 'Are you alright Madam?'...That's why I was struck, when I met you doctor, in the corridor and you smiled at me...Then when you asked me 'Madam, would you like to join in the consultation with your husband...I need your opinion' it didn't seem true..."

17.6 What Does the Psychosexologist Talk About?

The psychosexologist talks about many issues, but she/he will explore the emotionality of the patient and the partner for a short time. In those moments, neither the patient nor the partner is fully aware.

"Probably, at this moment you are confused and disorientated. Everything seems pointless except for fighting the disease. Bear in mind that you will never be alone and during and after treatment you will always be able to meet me: you can talk about your anxieties and fears, fears about the future or about sexuality. And if you feel that you are not the same as before...it is not necessarily the case that the 'after,' though different, will not be of a satisfactory quality..."

The patient's questions, in these moments, are few but clear..."How will my body change?" How will I feel after the treatment?

Case Illustration 5
His Voice

"I've never had a real relationship. Perhaps I've never been in love." Alex,43 "I don't have time for women, I said to myself and I always had relationships only for sex...with paid women mostly...high class obviously...well selected.... I won't deny that I would now like to have a companion just for me. Like my friend Michele. He had surgery on his knee and his girlfriend would visit him every day... she was sweet and tender... she brought him jam for breakfast the following morning... I don't like jam... but friends give you so much encouragement, affection, but they don't take care of you... Sometimes, I'm ashamed, I call my mother, just to hear her voice....

Case Illustration 6
Her Voice

"It's really difficult" Virginia, 41 "Sexuality has become a chore with David (her husband). One time he couldn't have an erection, another time he could but it didn't last long enough, another time he didn't want to... and it is not enough for him to be alive and well after that bad diagnosis. He takes drugs for impotence ... one time it works and another not ... And I always find myself understanding, understanding his frustration, not to be disappointed ... But frankly I would like to forget everything and start over again ....

17.7 Body Image, Fertility

Each patient answers these questions differently, and research has shown that survivors of orchidectomy between the ages of 32 and 35 (whether they had a prosthesis or not) reported that they did not feel less manly, unless the loss of a testicle hindered sexual performance.

Other studies however [5] show that 16% of survivors of testicular neoplasm experience deep concerns about the change in body image and the resulting feeling of vulnerability. Above all, they describe how embarrassed and anxious they are about the possibility that others might notice the missing testicle, asking them embarrassing questions like "What happened to you?" They also constantly feel different from other men.

In other studies on adult patients (over 40s), about a third of the survivors reported a decrease in physical attractiveness ("I look in the mirror and I don't see myself..."), as well as feeling less attractive.

Keep in Mind

Nevertheless, 52% of patients report having changed their body scheme significantly, but 89% of survivors' partners do not report any decreased physical or sexual interest in their partner.

"He has already suffered enough and I well know how important it is for him to once again feel desired, sought after, loved... When I had a nodule removed from my breast, I got over it on my own... He (the patient) gave me a lot of affection... but to feel like a new woman... I had to get strength and look for help... He without me... he would let himself go...

Furthermore, the evaluation of patients with testicular prosthesis implants (which also included a significant number of adolescents) in the long-term follow-ups shows significant improvements in the complaisant perception of their bodies (1 year after implantation) as well as greater self-esteem and confidence in conducting sexual intercourse [15].

17.8 What of Fertility?

Clinical studies have investigated this primarily in adult survivors and in the follow-ups, where the storage of semen after diagnosis and before each treatment (about 24% of patients) had safeguarded the possibility of parenthood.

On the other hand, the literature refers to reduced fertility in patients with azoospermia and with erectile dysfunction caused by psychosocial (or psychiatric) discomfort and permanent dry ejaculation [16].

For all other patients, it was noted that the average time from diagnosis to the birth of the first posttreatment child is about 7 years, depending on the type of treatment and assisted reproductive technique.

These reproductive procedures appear to affect 22% of couples with a patient who has survived the diagnosis of testicular neoplasm.

17.9 When Chemotherapy Is Introduced

That is not all.

Treatments for testicular cancer are often multidisciplinary. In addition to surgery and removal of the diseased testicle, cisplatin-based chemotherapy may be prescribed, depending on the neoplastic typology and the clinical phase of the tumor.

In such cases, the psychological burden on the patient and the partner should be further assessed. *The mutuality of the relationship can, if not psychosexually monitored, become a deterrent to patient compliance and quality of life after treatment.*

Keep in Mind

Cisplatin is a very aggressive chemotherapy treatment that can lead to disabling side effects:

1. Nausea and vomiting
2. Metallic flavor in the mouth
3. Bruises and blood loss from the nose
4. Fatigue and reduction of physical stamina
5. Fever and chills
6. Hair loss
7. Oral ulcers (on the mucous membrane of the mouth)
8. Hearing and balance disorders
9. Damage to lung parenchyma
10. In some cases, secondary neoplasms

These side effects and their adverse impact on both sexuality and quality of life in general affect 60% of patients.

Although most of these symptoms can be mitigated by additional ad hoc medication, long-term effects include mostly metabolic and circulatory disorders, peripheral nerve damage, and infertility.

This is the high price to be paid to achieve a 90% survival rate, offering the possibility of recovery even for patients with extensive metastases.

17.10 What of the Emotional and Psychological Price?

17.10.1 How Is the Lack of a New Motivation in Life Eased?

"…I take 12 different medications every day and I always wonder if it's worth it…" declares Arthur, 45 "…I vomited for months, I had to wear a wig, I couldn't eat or swallow and I didn't want to be seen by anyone….I felt like a piece of meat to be thrown away…I've suffered too much to save my skin…and even when they tell you that you are out of danger…it seems to you that you have paid too high a price to save your skin…Yeah…what skin? I don't know who I am anymore… everything is different and when I wake up in the morning, I feel so old… at least twenty years older…"

Take-Home Message

A study by Rieker et al. [17] clearly showed that survivors of testicular neoplasms suffer a profound and prolonged discomfort, compared to healthy subjects, even in the sexual sphere:

1. Ejaculation disorders 24%
2. Erection disor ders 10%
3. Sexual desire 11%
4. Sexual satisfaction 12%

Finally, patients who have received chemotherapy report worse problems of infertility and sexual dysfunction.

A further study by Tinkler et al. [18] analyzed the sexuality of patients with testicular seminoma who were treated with radiotherapy. Compared to the control group, they showed a decrease in libido, difficulty in maintaining an erection, minimal intensity of orgasm, and a reduction in the production of seminal fluid (poor or semidry ejaculation).

The result was a low frequency of sexual intercourse and little interest in sex, especially in patients around 35 years of age, compared to those of a more mature age. Younger patients, on the other hand, reported a tendency to good frequency and performance.

17.11 The Study and the Clinical Practice

This is not all.

Many studies, including Van Basten et al. [19], show that patients who have undergone several cycles of chemotherapy reported severe reduction in libido, disorders of excitation and orgasm, erectile dysfunction, poor ejaculation, and much more severe sexual disorders than patients treated with orchidectomy.

The same study added that Raynaud's phenomenon (angiopathy) was found in 32.7% of patients treated with chemotherapy.

Jonker-Pool et al. [20] stressed the role of psychological factors in sexual dysfunction, depending on the treatment suffered:

1. 22.5% of patients treated with orchidectomy had at least one type of sexual dysfunction.
2. 22% of patients treated with radiotherapy reported a decrease in libido and sexual frequency even for a low testosterone level. 14.5% reported erection disorders.

3. Patients who had undergone chemotherapy were consistent in reporting a 29.5% reduction in libido and a 28.5% reduction in orgasm.
4. A study shows how subjective psychological implications, the inability to satisfy the partner (22%), or the inhibition toward the partner (9.6%), together with the physical condition and the fear of a relapse, were conditioning and deterrent elements of intimacy.
5. In addition, in 15% of patients, changes in sexual functioning were already evident at the time of diagnosis, in 13.8% at the beginning of treatment, in 66% after treatment.

17.12 Sex and Marital Status

It is not irrelevant to note how influential the civil "status" of patients is in the study of sexual dysfunction after treatment, i.e., single or married? What is the difference in intimacy?

Single patients reported more sexual problems at diagnosis than married patients or patients with a fixed relationship, except with regard to sexual desire.

On the other hand, the partners felt more emotionally involved in affectively supporting the patient, filtering negative emotions, and supporting him in moments of hopelessness.

Singles, though, would seem deprived of this "protective" relationship, while admittedly enjoying the proximity of friends, they were more frightened by the risk of infertility and about future intimate relationships. Moreover, singles had sex with different partners, and the piecemeal nature of this frequency over time did not give them the feeling of a "safe and secure" perspective of the future.

Furthermore, anxiety-depressive symptoms or severe depression after chemotherapy was more frequent in single patients than in patients in a stable relationship, while 3 months after orchiectomy, single patients reported erection disorders and lower sexual satisfaction. One year after removal of the testicle, depressive symptoms in single patients had improved with the support of adequate medication therapy, but the quality of sexual intercourse still seemed dysfunctional.

Keep in Mind

This leads us to emphasize the "therapeutic" value of the couple in moments of post-traumatic stress and the "therapeutic alliance" with the clinical team.

This factor should also be valued more in the surgical context, considering the patient not only as a passive victim of the disease but as the solution and instrument of his own recovery.

<u>Daily clinical experience shows that even couples with relationship problems, at the time of diagnosis, declared an "armistice with the previous two-way conflict (diagnosis)," to reorganize the emotional energies into a "mutual survival."</u>

"We are going through a separation phase" declares Alice, Lucio's wife, 39 years old "and at this moment I can't even think about it...I realize that every previous malaise now seems like nonsense to me...Him, who never comes home before 9 p.m....who doesn't even ask you 'how are you?' always attached to the computer or iPhone for work ... not even a surgeon would ... and now I even feel that I miss those oddities ... I feel lost ... the idea that in the future I could be alone and not see him anymore ... terrifies me"....."

17.13 Body Workshop

But the couple acts as a secure "laboratory" to overcome also the change of body image which is internalized by the patient and the partner, before and after the diagnosis and treatment for testicular cancer.

How does the idea of him change when he looks in the mirror? And will she still feel attracted to her partner's body?

The study by Gritz et al. [10, 11] was the first to approach this issue, involving 34 couples who had shared the entire therapeutic process, from diagnosis through various treatments.

So far, clinical studies.

Take-Home Message

It was found that:

1. Almost all patients reported that the impact of the diagnosis had greatly altered their perception of their body image and their seductive capacity.
2. However, 64.7% of patients and partners (89%) did not report a lower degree of attraction to the other partner after treatment, although 36% of men felt less attractive than the perception of partners (12%).
3. Patients' perception of a loss of seductive capacity toward the partner was confirmed as a "long-term" condition, while the partner (12%) hypothesized it or perceived it from the patient's emotionality, as a temporary condition, caused by the pathology and consequent treatments.
4. Differently, patients who had undergone cisplatin treatment showed in 70% of cases a total loss of virile and seductive capacity toward the partners, also because these partners, in spite of themselves, had to emotionally support the partner for all treatment cycles (and collateral symptoms) more with a "nursing and maternal" role, and not as a "lover."
5. A final difference is found in the literature between couples already established at the time of diagnosis of testicular cancer and those formed after treatment. The former experienced more sexual satisfaction than the latter, although the partners of both groups reported less sexual satisfaction.
6. 12% of men and 22% of women in stable partnerships prior to diagnosis had more relational, clinical, and sexual problems after treatment.

Looking at these results, it is clear how the preliminary anamnesis of the couple's history or of the affective relationships of singles is essential when hypothesizing the real objectives of a recovery of the patient's quality of life after treatment, the different types of psychosexological counselling, according to sexual habits, and the presence of a fixed partner, of various partners, of homosexual partners.

"My partner is very frightened..." reflects Valerio, 31 "... after the orchiectomy, Stefano (the partner) has become more reticent...there's pampering, hugs...but he runs away from any kind of intimacy or sexual play...he has started 'chatting' (online) again...he goes out with friends....I think he sees someone else too...He says that it is a passing moment, that he has to recover from the shock...that he has never had indirect experiences of surgery before me...but...I remain perplexed, just...I just want someone to welcome me...last night I cried. Stefano was very worried. He told me 'don't be silly! You are a man...pull yourself together...' I just wanted to be accepted..."

17.14 When Does Post-traumatic Stress End?

This fragility is also a legacy of post-traumatic stress following diagnosis that according to a study by Dahl et al. [21] could continue even 11 years after diagnosis, as is well represented by specific research.

One thousand four hundred eighteen patients (diagnosed with testicular cancer 11 years earlier) responded to a questionnaire on post-traumatic symptoms—Impact of Event Scale (IES)—sent home and filled in at leisure:

- 4.5% of patients had 100% post-traumatic stress
- 6.4% had 60% post-traumatic stress
- 10.9% had 40% post-traumatic stress

with symptoms of anxiety, poor self-esteem, chronic fatigue, depression, sleep disorders, irritability, and apathy.

In conclusion, the study would seem to suggest that despite an excellent prognosis, testicular cancer leaves these patients with a long-term vulnerability that should be further investigated in follow-ups, not only relating to sexual response but in all areas of the patient's quality of life and emotional well-being.

Moreover, the study by Skaali et al. [22] also showed the negative effects of chemotherapy on patients with testicular cancer who reported fatigue, psychological discomfort, and cognitive problems. One hundred twenty-two patients undergoing orchidectomy and chemotherapy were evaluated 1 year after the end of treatment.

During the follow-up, questionnaires were administered on psychological discomfort, fatigue, peripheral neurotoxicity.

Patients were divided into three groups:

- Patients undergoing orchidectomy without chemotherapy
- Patients who had undergone a chemotherapy cycle
- Patients who had undergone multiple cycles of chemotherapy

The patients of the second and third groups showed progressive cognitive problems with strong psychological discomfort, anxiety in the confrontation with daily reality, disorganization in the time taken for personal hygiene or walking, fatigue, asthenia, deflection of mood.

Although these aspects do not directly form part of surgical treatment, specialists cannot fail to investigate concomitant and post-surgical treatment issues, especially when the invalidation of the patient sets him great limits in expressing himself in everyday life and in the progression of life.

Case Illustration 7

The Voice of...

"Giovanni is a professional actor" says Paolo, 35, his younger brother "The diagnosis has terrorized everyone in the family. Even if he doesn't admit it. He was hysterical. He only thought about rehearsals in the theatre, touring Italy, making his debut....

Even entering the operating room he insisted, 'Take the iPhone, you could call my agent to confirm the rehearsal days in the theatre' ...Giovanni always swims against the tide, he never looks at reality, he only ever sees his work ... I think it is his den where he can hide from life ... he hasn't had a relationship that's lasted more than three months....When he doesn't work...he becomes a grouchy, intolerant, moody old man who grumbles about everything...He's very alone, he only has me... We lost our parents in a road accident eight years ago...now we live together...two different lives...He always travels around the world...I work in the Bank every day... but we always keep in touch..."

Case Illustration 8

The Voice of....

"I met Vincent at the spa" recounts Arturo, 43 "We fell in love right away. He (Vincent) is younger...he's 35 years old and is a 'puppy to be led' ... "I'm his guardian-lover as he says ... but the diagnosis has changed our relationship. It is still very intimate, but Vincent betrays me whenever he can ... he says that they are not betrayals ... that it has nothing to do with me, his escape ... he says that I do not like him ... after surgery he feels different and wants to see if others also notice that he is less attractive ... He makes me suffer all this ... I do not know how to help him ....

Case Illustration 9

The Voice of…

"Martino was my university friend with whom I studied for 4 years" says Flavia, 32 "We are friends, bosom buddies... We also did the Erasmus together in Spain ....Often we are mistaken for lovers ... we laugh ... for me he is a brother ... I am an only child and I like this idea ... How pleased I was to accompany him today to the surgeon.

I know that he has to undergo surgery ... his parents were happy that I went with him ... they felt more relaxed ... but I don't know how to help him ... it seems strange to see myself here with him but I wouldn't have been able to work today ... tell me Doctor, the day of the surgery ... is it better that only the parents are present or should I be here too?

17.15 Conclusions

Saving the life of a patient is definitely the priority of the clinician and surgeon. That, though, is not enough. "The quality of life" is another basic aspect that the clinician cannot renounce out of respect and responsibility toward the patient.

A multidisciplinary approach can simplify this process of researching, adapting, and motivating post-traumatic stress, *firstly, by educating the patient to understand, in a simple way, the neurovegetative processes resulting from the removal of the testicle and motivating him to give a "blameless" meaning to the emotional states of discomfort and fatigue.* Emotional, sexual, social, and relational recoveries also depend very much on the therapeutic contract and on the clinical program agreed upon at diagnosis.

The patient must be aware that if during surgery he can but leave the "lifesaving" practice to the surgeon through the removal of a testicle, in the post-surgical period, it will only be up to himself, the partner, and the psychosexologist to deal with the neurological reorganization schedule: rhythms that will not coincide with the character traits and the will to resume "quickly and well" any type of activity and fluctuating rhythms that seem slow and not always salient, more productive in the morning, more tiring in the afternoon.

The healing process is also a form of self-learning, and the patient can enhance his own medical and life culture.

He understands that in the post-surgical period, he is the true protagonist of his own healing and the "raw material" to reinvest in a new man plan: skillful, efficient, capable of liking himself and of liking.

17.16 Self-Check Path

There are no right or wrong answers. It is just a way to reflect and to rethink our clinical approach and our reactions to a patient with testicular cancer.

1. When a patient shows clear signs of opposition to a chemotherapeutic treatment: do you think it is a big problem, do you entrust it to the psychosexologist to change his mind, do you ask for psychiatric advice, or do you try to listen to the patient's reasons?
2. If a young patient asks you a thousand questions about future sexuality and fertility and is single: do you postpone the problem until he has a fixed partner and recommend he relax, do you try to examine with the psychosexologist the quality of life of the patient, or do you postpone the matter until after the surgical treatment?
3. If a partner demonstrates a lot of perplexity about the treatment you recommend for the patient (husband): do you think that the partners are always a big problem to manage, do you consult with the psychosexologist about what to do, or do you leave the responsibility of the therapeutic choice to the patient and to the partner?
4. When you are in front of a homosexual patient: do you think this is a complication, do you approach the issue of treatment with great precision so as not to leave anything in abeyance, or do you think that the patient's sexuality is too singular and pretentious?
5. If the psychosexologist asks you for a little more time regarding an orchidectomy, arguing that the patient is too young and is not ready for treatment: do you think that the priority is to remove the tumor, do you try to understand the reasoning of the colleague, or do you organize a meeting with the patient, the family, and the psychosexologist to build a path that takes into account the patient's schedule and the surgical schedules?
6. *If during a follow-up you find that the patient does not enjoy a sexuality equal to the perspectives described by you: do you try to understand if the surgical intervention may have caused this unexpected outcome, do you think that it is only a psychological question of the patient, or do you advise him to talk to the psychosexologist and prescribe a pharmacological therapy for sexual function?*
7. *When the operating theatre is over, do you think:* "Finally I am free from fatigue and tension," "I hope that everything goes well without complications," "Before leaving the hospital, I'll pass on to see the patients in the ward"…

17.17 Medical History Questions

17.17.1 For the Patient

1. When you learned about the diagnosis, what did you think?
2. What do you fear most about this situation?
3. Do you feel supported by the surgeon and doctors you have met so far?
4. What did you understand the most about their explanations?
5. With regard to sexuality following treatment, what assurances and information have you received?
6. Has this diagnosis truncated any work or family project already in place?

7. Who knows about his problem?
8. Who has surprised you among friends, relatives, and partners for the support you are getting?
9. Who on the other hand disappointed you, showing less involvement than you expected?
10. Are you worried about your partner? Does she seem worried?
11. Does being single make your situation more difficult? Or do you feel that you can better manage the disease by taking care of yourself?

17.17.2 For the Partner

1. How do you think your partner is reacting?
2. Do you think he will have sufficient motivation to overcome the chemotherapy cycles?
3. What do you talk about most often?
4. What worries you most about your future?
5. Have you already dealt with complex clinical situations like this in the past?
6. Are you more concerned about the surgical treatment or the resumption of sexuality?
7. Have you told anyone about your concern? What did you expect from the other person? Affection, understanding, help?
8. Do you have children? Is it one of your projects to become parents?
9. Tell me what your future might look like after your surgical treatment?
10. How do your families of origin participate? Did you expect any further feedback?

17.17.3 For the Homosexual Partner

1. What did you think when you learned about your partner's diagnosis?
2. Has he told you something that you are sorry about during this time?
3. If he proposed ending the relationship for fear of not being attractive, how would you cope with this proposal?
4. What is most worrying about this situation?
5. Do you think you can follow your partner throughout the clinical path?
6. Who are the people closest to you at the moment?
7. If you had the opportunity to have sexual intercourse with other partners, would you experience this opportunity at this time as an escape from suffering or would you find yourself without desire?
8. How do you envisage a resumption of sexuality with your partner?
9. How long have you known each other? Has sexuality changed during your relationship?
10. What impressed you the most about the clinical procedure that was proposed to your partner?

References

1. Cullen JW et al (2007) Testicular cancer. In: Bleyer WA, Barr RD (eds) Cancer in adolescents and young adults. Springer, Berlin, pp 237–248
2. Bleyer A et al (2007) In: Bleyer WA, Barr RD (eds) Cancer in adolescents and young adults. Springer, Berlin, pp 1–26
3. Melissa Y et al (2010) Sexual and emotional relationships, body image, and fertility in young people and young adults who survived testicular cancer: a review of the literature. J Adolesc 47(2):115–125
4. Brodsky MS (1999) Impressions of testicular cancer survivors about the impact on their lives. Qual Health Res 5:78–96
5. Sheppard C et al (2001) An evaluation of sexual difficulties in men after treatment for testicular cancer. Sex Relat Ther 16:47–58
6. Tuinman MA et al (2006) Self-esteem, social support and mental health in testicular cancer survivors: a comparison based on relationship status. Urol Oncol 24:279–286
7. Rudberg L et al (2000) Health-related quality of life in survivors of testicular cancer 3-13 years after treatment. J Psychosoc Oncol 18:19–31
8. Tuinman MA et al (2005) Marital and sexual satisfaction in survivors of testicular cancer and their partners. Support Care Cancer 13:540–548
9. Caffo O et al (1999) Valutazione della vita sessuale dopo l'orchiectomia seguita dalla radioterapia per il primo stadio di ca del testicolo. BJU Int 83:462–468
10. Gritz ER et al (1989) Psycho-social conflict in long-term survivors of testicular cancer. J Psychosoc Oncol 6:41–63
11. Gritz ER et al (1989) Long-term effects of testicular cancer and sexual functioning in married couples. Cancer 64:1560–1567
12. Bancroft J et al (2009) The dual control model: current status and future prospects. J Sex Res 46:121–142
13. Wiechno P et al (2007) The quality of life and hormonal interference in testicular cancer survivors in the era of cisplatin. Eur Urol 52:1448–1455
14. Jonker PG et al (2004) Male sexuality following cancer treatment. Need for support: testicular cancer compared to malignant lymphoma. Patient Educ Couns 52:143–150
15. Turek PJ et al (2007) The testicular Prosthesis Study Group. J Urol 172:1427–1430
16. Drasga RE et al (1983) Fertility after chemotherapy for testicular cancer. J Clin Oncol 1:179–183
17. Rieker PP et al (1989) Psychosocial factors, behavioral therapies and results, a comparison between survivors to testicular cancer and a control group of healthy men. Cancer 64:2399–2407
18. Tinkler S et al (1992) Sexual morbidity following radiotherapy for testicular germ cell tumors. Radiother Oncol 25:207–212
19. Van Basten JP et al (1997) Sexual dysfunctions in patients with nonseminoma testicular cancer are chemotherapy-induced angiopathy-related. J Clin Oncol 15:2442–2448
20. Jonker Pool G et al (1997) Sexual functioning in patients with testicular cancer. Cancer 80(3):454–464
21. Dahl A et al (2016) Post traumatic aspect and long-term disorders of testicle cancer. J Cancer Surviv 10(5):842–849
22. Skaali T et al (2011) Cognitive problems reported by patients with testicular cancer: fatigue, psychological, neuropsychological performance. J Psychosom Res 70(5):403–410

Bibliography

Hanna NH, Einhorn LH (2014) Testicular cancer—discoveries and updates. N Engl J Med 371:2005–2016

Albers P et al (2015) Guidelines on testicular cancer: 2015 update. Eur Urol 68:1054–1068

Hanna N, Einhorn LH (2014) Testicular cancer: a reflection on 50 years of discovery. J Clin Oncol 32:3085–3092

Beyer J et al (2013) Maintaining success, reducing treatment burden, focusing on survivorship: highlights from the third European consensus conference on diagnosis and treatment of germ-cell cancer. Ann Oncol 24:878–888

Beard CJ et al (2015) Follow-up management of patients with testicular cancer: a multidisciplinary consensus-based approach. J Natl Compr Cancer Netw 13:811–822

McGlynn KA, Devesa SS, Sigurdson AJ, Brown LM, Tsao L, Tarone RE (2003) Trends in the incidence of testicular germ cell tumors in the United States. Cancer 97(1):63–70

Surgical and Radiological Correction of Varicocele in Infertile Male: Sexuality and Quality of Life

18

Elena Vittoria Longhi and Paolo Maria Michetti

18.1 Introduction

Varicocele is diagnosed in 15% of men, of whom 19–41% will have primary infertility and 45–81% secondary infertility. The alterations in testicular function derived from varicocele appear to be related to an increase in testicular temperature, with damaging effects on spermatogenesis and germ cells.

Growing evidence suggests, among other things, that the pathophysiology of varicocele could lead to partial dysfunction of the hypothalamic-pituitary-gonadal axis at the level of the Leydig cells and hormonal alteration [1]. Varicocelectomy would therefore improve the total serum testosterone level in >80% of patients and increase testicular size.

It should be noted that the incidence of varicocele increases with age (as with hypogonadism) as venous valves undergo changes with the gradual aging of their walls. In older patients who develop varicocele and hypogonadism, the benefit of varicocelectomy on serum testosterone levels is related to the age of the individual.

Men in the fifth and sixth decades of life who underwent low serum total testosterone varicocelectomy achieved as much improvement as younger men [2].

In this regard, another study Abdel-Meguid et al. [3] compared patients with varicocele and infertility who had undergone varicocelectomy, patients with varicocele who had not undergone any type of treatment, and finally normal individuals without varicocele and infertility.

At a 6-month follow-up, patients who had undergone varicocelectomy showed testosterone levels comparable to those of fertile men with varicocele. However, improved post-varicocelectomy testosterone levels had not reached levels comparable to those of healthy, fertile men without varicocele.

E. V. Longhi et al., *Psychosexual Counseling in Andrological Surgery*,
https://doi.org/10.1007/978-3-319-99646-2_18

This suggests that some damage to the testicles and testicular function may not be irreversible and early varicocelectomy may be very important for the quality of life of these patients. Many studies argue that men with varicocele and hypogonadism should be surgically repaired even when their future fertility is not in question.

18.2 Diagnosis and Surgical Treatment

Careful physical examination remains the primary method of varicocele detection. An obvious varicocele is often described as feeling like a bag of worms.

Keep in Mind
Varicoceles vary in size and can be classified into three degrees:

- Grade III: easily identified by inspection alone
- Grade II: identified by palpation without bearing down (Valsalva maneuver)
- Grade I: identified only by bearing down, which increases intra-abdominal pressure
- Subclinical: not detected on physical exam; found by ultrasounds or other imaging study

When the clinical examination findings are equivocal, high-resolution color-flow Doppler ultrasonography is the diagnostic method of choice. It defines a varicocele as a hollow tubular structure that grows following a Valsalva maneuver. The color of the signal identifies the blood flow and direction within the varicocele. The characteristic reverse flow of varicoceles is confirmed by prolonged flow augmentation within a colored flow area; the flow changes color (i.e., reverses) on real-time imaging.

Teenagers and Clinical Practice
The indications for repairing varicoceles in adolescents include the following:

- Palpable (especially grade III) left varicocele associated with decreased testicular size (with the volume of the left testis being at least 20% less than that of the right); palpable (especially grade III) varicocele with abnormal semen analysis results
- Large (grade III) symptomatic (painful) varicocele
- Bilaterally palpable varicocele with testicular atrophy

The indications in male partner of a couple attempting to conceive include the following:

- A varicocele is palpable (can be felt).
- The male partner has one or more abnormal semen parameters or sperm function test results.
- The couple has documented infertility.
- The female partner has normal fertility or potentially correctable infertility.

The primary form of treatment for varicoceles is surgery. The goal of varicocele treatment is to stop the backward flow of blood from the abdomen to the scrotum with high success, preservation of arterial flow to the testis, and the minimization of patient discomfort and morbidity. There are several ways to treat varicoceles, including radiographic obliteration and surgical repair of various approaches, and the efficacy of the techniques is nearly equivalent.

The most common surgical approaches are inguinal, retroperitoneal (abdominal), and subinguinal.

Inguinal ligation is achieved by incising the inguinal canal down to the external inguinal ring.

After cord isolation, the testicular artery is preserved, and the veins of the cord are ligated and divided.

18.3 Subinguinal Microsurgical Varicocelectomy

Subinguinal microsurgical varicocelectomy is currently a popular approach. It has the advantage of allowing the spermatic cord structures to be pulled up and out of the wound so that the testicular artery, lymphatics, and small periarterial veins may be more easily identified.

The access is achieved through an incision at or near the pubic tubercle that obviates the opening of the external oblique aponeurosis. The advantages of subinguinal varicocele ligation include decreased pain and easier access to the spermatic cord, especially among obese men and those with a history of inguinal surgery.

The retroperitoneal approach offers great proximal control of the spermatic vein near its insertion at the renal vein, and this approach may be accomplished also laparoscopically. High retroperitoneal ligation of varicocele, also known as the Palomo technique, is performed through a horizontal incision medial and inferior to the ipsilateral anterior superior iliac spine and extending medially. The external oblique fascia is incised in the direction of the fibers and the internal oblique muscle retracted cranially to expose the internal spermatic veins proximal to the internal inguinal ring.

18.4 Surgical Approach in Sequence

An informed consent must be obtained before performing every kind of approach. Patient should be informed about possible complications after surgery—infection, bleeding, 5–10% of recurrent varicocele, 2–5% chance of developing a hydrocele, and 0.9% of injury to the testicular artery with possible testicular atrophy—and about alternative to the proposed procedure and the related risks.

The treatment of varicocele by percutaneous embolization of the internal spermatic vein is a safe and effective minimally invasive procedure.

Its very low morbidity and complication rates, high long-term success rates, and demonstrated cost effectiveness relative to surgery have led some authors to argue that percutaneous embolic techniques should be the primary therapy to treat varicoceles or at least a viable and valuable alternative to surgical options.

The internal spermatic vein is accessed primarily via cannulation of the femoral or brachial vein through a retrograde approach with subsequent balloon and/or coil occlusion of the varicocele. The advantages of percutaneous embolization include preservation of the testicular artery and the relatively noninvasive nature of the technique.

Take-Home Message

However, the percutaneous approach can be fraught with troublesome access to the vein, and postoperative complications such as contrast allergies, arterial injury, thrombophlebitis, and coil migration are uncommon but tangible risks. This approach is often reserved for recurrent varicoceles after open surgical repair.

18.5 Varicocele and Sexual Disorders

18.5.1 Having Said That, What Kind of Sexuality Do These Patients Enjoy?

Keep in Mind

Very few studies have evaluated the association between varicocele and erectile dysfunction (ED). A study by Keller et al. [4] included 32,856 clinical cases and 98,568 follow-ups. Among the patients sampled, 3.3% had a diagnosis of varicocele followed by surgical treatment, while 1.2% had no treatment for the same disease. Research results showed that patients with varicocele who underwent varicocelectomy reported less discomfort with erectile response and its maintenance during the sexual act.

That is not all. Lotti et al. [5] evaluated the impact of varicocele on overall sexual function (study 1—2448 patients with an average age of 52 years) and the possible association between varicocele and prostatitis (study 2—139 patients with an average age of 38 years).

In study 1, varicocele was clinically classified into three grades according to the Dubin criteria. Several hormonal parameters were also evaluated. All patients in study 2 underwent simultaneous color scrub and transrectal color Doppler ultrasound (CDU) together with seminal and interleukin-8 characteristics, a surrogate marker of prostatitis.

18.6 The Statistical Results

After adjustment for age, subjects with severe varicocele ($N = 284$, 11.6%, Dubin grades II and III) showed a reduction in testicular volume ($P < 0.01$), higher luteinizing hormone (LH) ($P < 0.05$), follicle-stimulating hormone (FSH) ($P < 0.0001$), and prolactin ($P < 0.05$) levels and also an enlarged or tender prostate in the digital-retrorectal examination ($P < 0.05$). Early ejaculation was the only sexual symptom significantly associated with varicocele (29.2% vs. 24.9% in subjects with or without varicocele, respectively, $P < 0.05$). In study 2, subjects with severe ultrasound defined varicocele (basal venous reflux increasing or not after the Valsalva maneuver, $N = 28$, 20.1%) showed CDU characteristics of prostatitis and higher levels of seminal interleukin-8. The presence of any degree of varicocele ($N = 40$, 28.8%) was also associated with symptoms of prostatitis, as measured by the score of the National Institutes of Health Chronic Prostatitis Symptom Index ($P < 0.05$), and in particular with the domain of pain ($P < 0.05$).

Take-Home Message

In conclusion, signs and symptoms of prostatitis are more common in patients with varicocele, who most often complain of premature ejaculation.

In addition, Zohdy et al. [6] reported that 60–70% of men with varicocele and infertility also reported hypoactive sexual desire, clinically associated with low serum testosterone levels (associated with varicocele).

18.7 Only Science or Also Psyche?

Why not also take into account the impact of infertility on sexual desire and the response to it? Why not also think about the conditioning generated by the hypothalamic-pituitary-gonadal axis, as mentioned in the beginning?

Daily clinical psychosexual experience often brings one into contact with patients who are humiliated and disappointed by their virility, saddened by the difficulty of not always giving pleasure to their partner and, above all, with a sense of guilt about a fertility that does not match the wishes of the couple.

Varicocelectomy certainly improves physical condition, but it increases the patient's magical expectations of unfettered sexuality, and when the relationships are unsatisfactory and unhealthy for the couple, the "emotional impotence" of the patient provokes anxiety, frustration, fear of losing the partner, and the fear of abandonment.

Although statistics indicate a high rate of assisted insemination births, many patients after varicocelectomy feel overwhelmed by these "genetic techniques" and lose the sense of playful sexuality with their partner.

Defeated in terms of sexuality and fertility, many patients suffer from hypoactive desire, difficulty with erections, and arousal.

Case 1

"I thought that after the surgery I would come back a new man" Lucien, 43 "Straight away things seemed to be back to their best…I didn't have much desire but…to please Francesca (his wife, 37) I tried and sometimes it was fine (sexual intercourse)…other times, it was better not to insist.

Then Francesca began to tell me that it was better to hurry up and try for a baby…. I was very keen too…but from there I lost control of sexual intercourse…I would sweat, I ejaculated as soon as Francesca touched me…I was constantly anguished…until Francesca…one evening, she made a scene… threatening to leave…Coming to you Doctor (psychosexologist) really is my last chance…"

Case 2

"I'm really discouraged" begins Laura, 34 "Riccardo (her husband, 42) has always made me anxious. First, his sexual inexperience (he had never had complete sexual intercourse…), then varicocele, surgical intervention…and now we are back at the beginning. He never takes the initiative and if one in every five attempts at sexual intercourse goes all the way we're lucky…He knows that I want a child so much. I even had a gastric tube fitted in order to lose 20 kg…the gynaecologist said that it was better to lose all that weight… so if I had to choose an assisted fertilization…why is it so easy for the other couples?"

Moreover, the treatment of varicocele is not necessarily recommended for all infertile men (with varicocele), and the current guidelines suggest some criteria for selecting candidates for surgical or radiological treatments.

Male Infertility Best Practice Policy Committee of the American Urological Association and the Practice Committee of the American Society for Reproductive Medicine has established the following criteria [7]:

1. The varicocele must be palpable on objective examination of the scrotum.
2. The couple has a known infertility.
3. The partner has a normal fertility or a potentially treatable cause of infertility.
4. The partner has abnormal sperm parameters or abnormal results on sperm function tests.

To these, the guidelines of the European Association of Urology (2012–2013) have included three other recommendations [8]:

1. The treatment of varicocele is recommended for adolescents with progressive testicular insufficiency, documented by clinical examinations.
2. No evidence indicates the benefit of varicocele treatment in infertile men who have normal sperm analysis or in men with subclinical varicocele.
3. The repair of varicocele should be considered in the case of clinical varicocele, oligospermia, duration of infertility >2 years, and otherwise unexplained infertility in the couple.

18.8 Varicocelectomy or Radiotherapy: Comparative Studies

Do we have clear scientific findings on the efficacy of treating varicocele with surgery or radiotherapy? Unfortunately, clinical studies have so far reported conflicting data with success and complication indices.

The study by Diegidio et al. [9] showed that the lowest relapse rate comes from the subinguinal microsurgical technique (2.7%), followed by the microsurgical inguinal technique with 9.7%, 12.5% with the Palomo technique, 4.29% with radiological embolization, 15.65% with the conventional inguinal technique, and 11.11% with laparoscopic intervention.

Finally, there is no lack of criticism and concern about the rates of recurrence after radiological embolization, which may be much higher than those that have so far come to light [10].

The impact of varicocele on sperm testing, on fertility, and, more recently, on premature ejaculation and miscarriage in partners has been investigated. In this retrospective study, four parameters (semen analysis, fertility, premature ejaculation, and partner miscarriage) were evaluated in relation to varicocele and varicocelectomy over a period of 13 years.

A total of 1711 patients with varicocele underwent varicocelectomy by the high inguinal method (251 cases), the subinguinal method (1375 cases), the scrotal method (34 cases), and the subinguinal method under local anesthesia (38 cases). The sperm count, motility, and morphology increased 3 months after surgery in 55%, 51%, and 46%, respectively (*P* values 0.000, 0.000, and 0.015, for each of the observed groups). Paternity was 56% after a year of follow-up post-varicocelectomy. Only 7 out of 82 azoospermic men had better sperm values after varicocelectomy, and only 1 of them with mild spermatogenic hypoplasia became a father.

The rate of miscarriage among the interviewees' partners was 59%. Early ejaculation improved in 75% of respondents.

Keep in Mind

In conclusion, varicocelectomy may not improve sperm parameters in all men, but it may improve the pregnancy rate, premature ejaculation and scrotal pain.

Furthermore, severe azoospermia and oligozoospermia have been reported between 4.3 and 13.3% in men with varicocele [11]. Existing data suggest that patients with nonobstructive azoospermia and clinical varicocele can improve seminal parameters after surgical repair of varicocele, and the possibility of improvement refers to histopathological testicular diagnosis [12]. Nevertheless, most studies that evaluated varicocele repair results in this category of patients did not include a control group, thus limiting conclusions on the benefits of performing varicocelectomy in patients with clinical varicocele [13].

18.9 Varicocele Relapse

There is more. The recurrence of varicocele is one of the most common complications associated mainly with the surgical technique used. The highest failure rates seem to be attributable (as the scientific literature shows) to inguinal varicocelectomy or macroscopic subinguinal varicocelectomy due to internal sperm veins which after surgical treatment dilate and cause relapses, whereas the highest incidence of recurrence observed with the retroperitoneal or laparoscopic approach would seem to be attributable to the inability to bind the external sperm vein or the (external) gonads [14].

Keep in Mind

It is the common opinion of researchers that the main reason for relapse is the presence of branched sperm veins that were not bound during the initial repair. In addition, see Al-Kandari et al. [15].

1. *Current evidence suggests that the initial treatment method most likely to cause relapses in an infertile man with a clinical varicocele is subinguinal varicocelectomy or microsurgical inguinal* [16].
2. *The recurrence of varicocele would appear more commonly caused by branches of internal sperm veins that had not initially been bound.*
3. *Treatment of relapse is only guaranteed in patients with clinical relapse who remain infertile or symptomatic* [17].

18.10 Costs and Benefits: Mind, Psyche, and Intimacy

In all of this, "how and to what extent does it affect the patient and the sexuality of the couple?

Although the study by Masson et al. [18] suggests that varicocele correction is a cheaper therapeutic modality than intrauterine insemination (IUI) and in vitro fertilization (IVF), daily clinical experience shows that the "emotional costs" for the patient and the couple often outweigh the benefit of surgical varicocelectomy or radiographic venous embolization.

A Chinese study by Niu et al. (2013) evaluated the psychological status of 110 patients with infertility and varicocele using the hospital anxiety and depression scale (HADS). The research then recruited 61 fertile "healthy" men of the same age (without diagnosis of varicocele).

Case Illustration 3

His Voice

"I was really lucky with the varicocele" begins Daniel, 28 "my twin brother Angelo however was really unlucky…Same surgeon, same medical team and we met you Doctor (psychosexologist)….I tell you frankly that at the beginning when you made me reflect on the possibilities of a complication…it made me anxious…but fortunately you did it with me and Angelo… everything we discussed with you happened to him...*recurrence, fear of pain, feelings of anxiety and loneliness on being discharged...I watched the film on anxiety and pelvic pain for the whole week after my discharge...but I remembered your words Doctor and trusted your story...Angelo had all the symptoms in the book...and also the relapse...I'm glad that he speaks to you...also this time...he doesn't listen to anyone at home...he doesn't talk to me either…'he's like a cat: when it's ill, it curls up into itself, it isolates itself and licks its wounds'…But he's talking to you, Doctor, right?*

It was found that anxiety rates in patients in the first group reached 62% while rates for depression reached 40% compared to 6% for anxiety and 4% for depression in the control group.

The researchers hypothesized that these percentages derived, in the hospital context, from the frequency of clinical examinations, visits of the medical team, and the intensity of testicular disorders.

But outside of the clinical context, anxiety and depression increase for the patient and the partner due to the fear of relapse, the lack of easily accessible medical references (" the surgeon has given us the direct number of the department, but the line is always busy and you cannot talk to anyone ….") , and an excess of optimism at the time of discharge "He is healed, in a few days he will be in shape…," due to a psychological process of infantilism of the patient who does not feel he is sufficiently cared for, due to the level of pain, due to the fear of taking too many painkilling drugs orally, due to the fear of not "being the same man as before"…

Case Illustration 4

His Voice

"Clarissa (his partner, 29) is very concerned" reports Claudio, 31 "Before me she had partner with erectile dysfunction or with little sexual experience. Now I have been diagnosed with varicocele and she has collapsed emotionally…She says that she feels persecuted by fate and that 'all men are incapable' of meeting her needs…" "(the psychosexologist) It does not seem very nice to me this thought, but surely Clarissa is in trouble…maybe she is showing her inadequacy…She is afraid of losing you …" "You know Doctor that just last night she told me 'Now you'll have an excuse to tell me that you are leaving me and that you can not make plans with me'…What can I do? "(psychosexologist) Tell her (Clarissa), please, on my part, that I need her information as a partner…and that if you agree, I would be happy to meet her with you Claudio…If instead Clarissa does not feel like it, for any reason, tell her that, there is no problem,…you love her the same… and will you (the patient) come again…" "I think that I will come" concludes Claudio "I was pushed by Clarissa herself to talk to you (psychosexologist) after Dr.…(surgeon) described how you work in the team….

The psychosexologist cannot work miracles, and the medical team does not expect this specialist to solve all the problems. If, however, a psychosexological service of accompaniment to the patient and partner is provided, even before the treatment chosen for varicocele, the less welcome events are also hypothesized:

"What would happen if you were soon faced with a relapse? How would your emotional commitment change if you knew you were to take this risk? Which of you would be less ready for such an eventuality?"

These questions make the patient more objective in the face of treatment and help him to underplay all kinds of magical expectations. Certainly, surgery and radiotherapy are carried out with the utmost care, but an unexpected complication or mishap may occur even months after treatment.

Making the patient and partner aware of various hypotheses of healing and/or relapse, lowering the level of anxiety and depression symptoms, better organizing emotional and psychological resources, preparing the couple for a more interactive collaboration with the medical team.

Case Illustration 5
Her Voice

"*...we were deluded that everything had gone well...*" *says Elisa, 42* "*Gianni (her husband, 36) seemed to react as the surgeon had said... He felt good, he had regained sexual desire....6 years of difference are a lot for a woman's body...and often I could not reach orgasm, just because I thought he might want a younger woman...Now (six months after varicocelectomy) it is I who have to reassure him every time he tries a sexual rapport...he says he is worried, he easily loses his erection...yet during the preliminaries he seems to react normally...*"

Case Illustration 6
Her Voice

"*I had planned with my gynaecologist to proceed with an intrauterine fertilization...*" *says Paola, 32* "*Pietro (the companion, 38) had been infertile and then with that varicocele...I had lost all hope of being able to become a mother 'normally'... He surprised me when he told me 'I'll have the operation, so then everything will go as you want....' We didn't take this decision lightly...we asked for more medical consultations...but we didn't think of a relapse one year after the first treatment... Pietro was discouraged...and I started thinking of proceeding with my gynaecologist...it was a pity that I wasted a year and a half...*"

Case Illustration 7
Her Voice

"*I was full of joy when I saw the positive pregnancy test...*" *says Clara, 39* "*Francesco had undergone treatment for varicocele and I didn't think that within 9 months of treatment I would become pregnant....Maybe it was a coincidence,...after treatment he had started to ejaculate early....Every time we tried a rapport was a disappointment...once he even ejaculated during foreplay...Now I'm in the 5th month of pregnancy...and we're happy...I hope that after the birth of the child...Francesco will come back to 'normal...as always'...(with a suitable sexual response)...Is that possible? Or am I deluding myself?*

We should then realize that the age of these patients, 13–45 years old, for example, is associated with complex relationships with family members or partners, who are helpless in the face of a loved one who, in any case, in order to be healed, will be "physically injured", as explained in the introductory chapters.

"I feel bad just thinking that they will hurt him and cut him right there....in the most delicate part of the organ..." "The wound won't be deep, will it Doctor?" "will he feel very bad?...

Voices of mothers, partners, and fathers who place themselves in the hands of surgeons and who, in the hope that everything goes for the best, can only worry, anxious, sometimes appearing petulant, or obsessive..., filling the waiting time... until the voice of the surgeon, smiling, announces ... "the treatment is successful!"

18.11 Conclusions

The complexity of varicocele treatment and the scientific discussions on the effectiveness of individual treatments lead us not only to investigate issues such as the impact of surgery or radiotherapy on the quality of life of the patient but also the opportunity of multidisciplinary interventions to educate the individual and the partner to the role of co-protagonists of care and not of passive patients.

Sexual handicaps, such as erectile dysfunction and arousal disorder, are just two of the clinical and emotional aspects of the patient after the trauma of varicocele treatment. Often solved clinically but not completely overcome at the psychological level by the patient who, unsure of his virility, competes with himself for fear of not reproducing a sexual response which is satisfactory to himself and his partner, sexuality thus becomes the legacy of a "violated" virility that must each time prove itself to be equal to the role.

18.12 Self-Check Path

A moment of self-assessment can be useful for every clinician to verify their aptitudes, their communicative style with the patient, and their approach to the various pathologies for which they are responsible.

1. A patient affected by the diagnosis of varicocele relapse is a therapeutic failure, a foreseen possibility, or an opportunity to review the therapeutic contract with the patient.
2. A young 20-year-old with varicocele who declares his phobia for blood, syringes needles, and pain is a spoiled patient, a case for the psychosexologist, a patient to be welcomed with great tranquility.
3. A patient with varicocele who asks you in detail about the surgical technique for the treatment of the disease, having searched through the internet: annoys you, makes the meeting more interesting, or you tell your colleagues and the psychosexologist that "it is a difficult patient."

4. The treatment of varicocele is, for you, a routine treatment, an insidious pathology, a treatment like so many others.
5. The age of the patient is an insignificant variable, a variable of no little importance, a component of the diagnosis.
6. What strikes you about the varicocele patient's interviews with the psychosexologist? That he is not a psychiatric patient, that he is complaisant, and that he has not suffered any physical or sexual trauma.
7. The relationship with the psychosexologist is routine, it is an exception, it frees you from the all too extensive stories of the patients, and it is a complementary consultation.

18.13 Medical History Questions

18.13.1 For the Patient

1. When you came to visit Dr…(surgeon), did you imagine you would have to undergo treatment?
2. Have you already undergone any other surgery?
3. What do you fear the most from admission to hospital to discharge?
4. What about from the discharge onwards?
5. How has your partner reacted so far?
6. Did you expect this reaction? Have there been any other situations in which the partner has acted in the same way?
7. What do you fear about the resumption of sexuality?
8. Do you have any specific questions you would like to ask me?
9. If you cannot become a parent, how will your future change?
10. What do you expect to be positive and less positive about this treatment?

18.13.2 For the Partner

1. How does your partner seem right now? After learning about the diagnosis of varicocele, did he seem different? (Was his behavior, anxious, worried…)
2. What sensations did you experience when faced with the diagnosis?
3. Are you more worried about your partner's varicocele or infertility?
4. How would your idea of a couple change if you could not become a mother?
5. Which of you wants to become a parent?
6. How would you rate your sexuality as a couple in the last year?
7. Have you ever undergone any gynecological surgery?
8. What do you feel when you think your partner will be treated in the genital area?
9. Do you think you will find it difficult to resume sexuality with your partner after treatment?
10. What concerns you most about your partner's varicocele treatment?

References

1. Li F et al (2012) Effect of surgical repair on testosterone production in infertile men with varicocele. Int J Urol 19:149–154
2. Hsiao W et al (2011) Older age is associated with similar improvements in semen parameters and testosterone after subinguinal microsurgical varicocelectomy. J Urol 185:620–625
3. Abdel-Meguid TA et al (2014) Effects of varicocele on serum testosterone and changes of testosterone after varicocelectomy: a prospective controlled study. Urology 84:1081–1087
4. Keller JJ et al (2012) Varicocele is associated with erectile dysfunction: a population-based case-control study. J Sex Med 9:1745–1752
5. Lotti F et al (2009) The association between varicocele, premature ejaculation and prostatitis symptoms: possible mechanisms. J Sex Med 6:2878–2887
6. Zohdy W et al (2011) Impact of varicocelectomy on gonadal and erectile functions in men with hypogonadism and infertility. J Sex Med 8:885–893
7. The Committee on policy best practices for male infertility of the American Urological Association and the Practice Committee of the American Society for Reproductive Medicine (2004) Report on varicocele and infertility. Fertil Steril 82(suppl 1):S142–S145
8. Jungwirth A et al (2012) Guidelines of the European Association of Urology on male infertility: 2012 update. Eur Urol 62:324–332
9. Diegidio P et al (2011) Overview of current techniques of varicocelectomy and their outcomes. BJU Int 108:1157–1172
10. Golstein M (2012) Surgical management of male infertility. In: Wein AJ et al (eds) Campbell-Walsh urology, 10th edn. Saunders, Philadelphia, pp 678–687
11. Czaplicki M, Bablok L, Janczewski Z (1979) Varicocelectomy in aozospermic patients. Arch Androl 3:51–55
12. Agger P, Johnsen SG (1978) Quantitative evaluation of testicular biopsies in varicocele. Fertil Steril 29:52–57
13. Esteves SC, Glina S (2005) Microsurgical varicocele repair recovery of spermatogenesis in men with azoospermia after subinguinal based on testicular histology. Int Braz J Urol 31:541–548
14. Collsaet et al (1980) The varicocele syndrome: venography determining the optimal level for surgical management. J Urol 124:833–839
15. Al-Kandari AM et al (2007) Comparison of outcomes of different varicocelectomy techniques: open inguinal, laparoscopic and subinguinal microscopic varicocelectomy: a randomized clinical trial. Urology 69:417–420
16. Chen SS et al (2014) Successful predictors of recurrent varicocele in infertile males with varicocelectomy. Andrology 46:738–743
17. Moon KH et al (2007) Recurrent varicoceles: causes and treatment using angiography and magnification assisted subinguinal varicocelectomy. Yonsei Med J 53:723–728
18. Masson P et al (2014) The varicocele. Urol Clin North Am 41(1):129–144

Bibliography

Baazeem A, Belzile E, Ciampi A, Dohle G, Jarvi K, Salonia A, Weidnerf W, Zini A (2011) Varicocele and male factor infertility treatment: a new meta-analysis and review of the role of varicocele repair. Eur Urol 60(4):796–808

Choi WS, Kim SW (2013) Current issues in varicocele management: a review. World J Mens Health 31(1):12–20

19 Penile Prosthesis Implant Following Pelvic Surgery

Elena Vittoria Longhi and Fulvio Colombo

19.1 Introduction

The surgical removal of tumors of the pelvis, due to the inadvertent damage of the hypogastric nerves and/or the pudendal blood vessels, can cause different degrees of postoperative erectile dysfunction.

The operations that most frequently can interfere with the erectile function are:

- Radical prostatectomy (RP), for localized prostate cancer
- Radical cystectomy (RC), for bladder cancer
- Abdominoperineal (AP) resection, for lower colon and rectal cancer
- Total pelvic exenteration, for large neoplasm of the colon

Furthermore, additional surgical operations involving the retroperitoneum may cause adverse effects on other male sexual functions as, for example, anejaculation (the so-called dry orgasm) that is the consequence of injuries of the nerves that come from the spine and are responsible for the emission of sperm.

19.2 The Surgical Approach

Operations at more risk for this kind of postoperative problems are:

- Retroperitoneal lymph node dissection, for testicular cancer
- AP resection, for colorectal cancer

For what the postoperative erectile function concerns, once released from the neoplasm, men usually have only partial erections, with the penis not rigid enough

E. V. Longhi et al., *Psychosexual Counseling in Andrological Surgery*,
https://doi.org/10.1007/978-3-319-99646-2_19

for penetration. Obviously, patients are more likely to recover erections when nerves on both sides of the prostate have been spared.

Moreover, the process of healing and growth of new blood vessels, which may contribute to restore an adequate blood flow to the penis, takes time to happen, and this fact could explain the delay in the return of erections.

In some cases, the recovery of the full functionality has been reported after 2 years from surgery.

According to the data of literature, at least 15% of men undergoing standard surgery to remove the bladder or prostate will recover full erections. We know that the age of patient at time of surgery plays a relevant role in the possibility to restore a complete penetration ability, since men under 50 are more likely to obtain full erections after operation.

Keep in Mind

Obviously, also the quality of patient's erections before surgery is a relevant point to predict his future possibility of erectile function recovery. In the literature, there are no definitive data about the impact of the different surgical techniques used during pelvic surgery (intra-fascial vs. inter- or extra-fascial techniques) on the erectile function recovery. Similarly, we have not yet incontrovertible information about the alleged greater reliability of robot-assisted laparoscopic technique compared to traditional open surgery, although increasing evidences seem to lead toward this direction.

19.3 The Erectile Function

Following the operation, many tools have been proposed to realize the so-called penile rehabilitation. The general aim is that of keeping cavernosal tissue healthy, thus counteracting the fibrosis process, which would make the chance of recovering erectile function very unlikely.

In case of successful sparing of the neurovascular bundle, at least on one side of the prostate, the administration of phosphodiesterase inhibitors (PDE5i—tadalafil, sildenafil, vardenafil, avanafil) can be effective.

Other kinds of treatment include intra-urethral creams, penile injections, and vacuum devices.

If these less invasive options resulted ineffective or are not suitable for the patient, the implantation of penile prosthesis is the only solution to allow the patient to recover the ability to penetrate.

There is strong evidence in the literature that supports the high level of satisfaction rate (when compared with PDE5-Is or ICI) reported by patients treated with RP and penile implants. Numbers of meta-analysis demonstrate the low complication rate and excellent mechanical reliability now achieved by these devices.

Keep in Mind

Interestingly, despite these encouraging data, it was found that the penile implant utilization rate is very low among patients undergoing RP, being of 2.3% (95% CI, 2.1–2.6). Possible explications of the low IPP utilization could be the improvement of surgical nerve-sparing techniques, the availability of effective nonsurgical treatment modalities (mainly PDE5i), and patient's reluctance to undergo surgery and concerns about PP.

Available data indicate the importance of psychological support to the implanted patient, in order to reduce his feeling of lack of sexual spontaneity and facilitate the psychosexual adaptation after surgery increasing patient satisfaction.

The degree of satisfaction following IPP implant seems to be related to many factors such as age of patient and partner, preoperative disease status, adjuvant cancer treatments, quality of preoperative erectile function, level of sexual activity, response to medical treatments for erectile dysfunction, partner's sexual function or dysfunction, lack of partner's support, partner's disinterest in sexual activity, and partner's fear of surgery.

For all these reasons, it is mandatory to offer to the patients who underwent pelvic surgery an effective multimodal support, in terms of "organic treatment" but also of psychological and sexual counseling, devoting full attention to expectations and actual needs and desires.

19.4 The Psychosexual Approach

Pelvic surgery involves a complex approach for both the specialist and the patient.

The patient and the partner mark the calendar (for several months) through the visits for the rehabilitation for incontinence, psychophysical disorders, and the resumption of sexuality with no inconsiderable variables. For example, orgasm without ejaculation for prostatectomized patients (who experience dry orgasm with retrograde ejaculation in the bladder).

Take-Home Message

This example alone shows us how the patient's "physical change" affects his or her quality of life for about 6–12 months, resulting in frustration, depression, chronic fatigue, and the idea of "no longer being the man he was before."

So when it comes to the hypothesis of a penile implant, the patient has experienced about a year oral therapy, intracavernous injection therapy, exercises using a vacuum devise (for the rehabilitation of the penis), and finally, with disillusionment and frustration, another procedure for a penile prosthesis.

A definitive intervention that puts an end to erectile dysfunction.

But at what emotional, psychological, intrapsychic, and social cost?
In detail:

19.5 Post-traumatic Chronic Stress (PSTD) and Psychophysical Consequences

The urologic oncological patient subjected to chronic post-traumatic stress (PSTD) presents clinical, neurological, and rehabilitation problems.

It has now been ascertained by the scientific community that from the moment of oncological diagnosis, the patient enters the process of general adaptation to clinical stress.

Broken down into:

- Alarm phase (diagnosis, stressor of life-threatening illness)
- Recognition phase (awareness of the danger to life)
- Resistance phase (with hyper-activation of the hypothalamic-pituitary-adrenal (HPA) axis)

Some studies have shown, using a sample of 120 patients with breast cancer, how the stress of a life-threatening disease alters, for example, the activity of NK cells and that only a high level of social, neurological, and sexual rehabilitation corresponds to an increased activity of NK cells and effective control of the tumor.

This parameter, expanded to all tumor themes, shows how it is necessary to involve several specialists who determine the priorities of intervention "on the patient," each time building a personalized treatment.

In particular, uro-sexual rehabilitation works on sexual rehabilitation (awareness of the physical and sexual maturity of the patient and partner), on continence (urological exercises of the pelvic floor), and on accompanying the patient with a neo-bladder and with an ostomy (in case of cystectomy with urinary deviation).

It is understood that the urologic oncological surgical team needs, as does the andrological surgical team, specialists in neuro-urology and neuro-sexology and an andrologist for pharmacological therapies for the resumption of erectile function.

Is though the resumption of the erectile response enough to assume that the urological oncological patient and partner will resume a satisfactory and lasting sexuality?

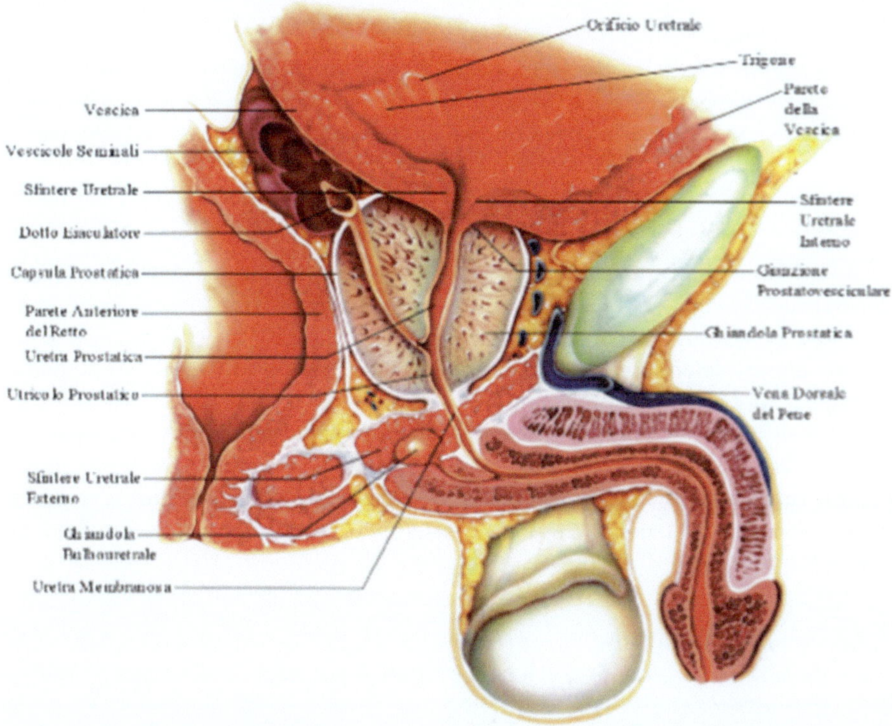

19.6 The Central Nervous System

Recent studies have emphasized the differences between acute stress (waiting for surgery, [1]) and chronic stress (the clinical process from the diagnostic phase to post-surgical rehabilitation to the perception of a new quality of life, [2]), as well as the importance of organizing an appropriate and effective response.

The activation of stress would therefore begin with the perception and recognition of the stressful event by the central nervous system (CNS), on which, among other things, depend the urological and sexual responses, which, just as for pain stimuli, initiate changes that would not be strictly related to the stressor (diagnosis).

The type of response according to the circuits followed by the stressor and more precisely on their ability to access the hypothalamus nucleus directly or indirectly has been described. Just as hypothesized that prolonged, stressful situations can be followed by the development of cognitive and emotional disorders.

Keep in Mind

Patients with chronic post-traumatic stress undergo biological processes triggered by the activation of the hypothalamic-pituitary-adrenal axis, with an alteration in the secretion of hormones, in the response of the autonomic nervous system, in the immune responses, in sleep disruption, and in the altered perception of symptoms and pain.

As well as altered emotional management (anxiety, depression, and panic attacks due to excessive cortisol production by the hippocampus).

These symptoms, associated with the reduced capacity to process and control fear reactions, determine in the patient and in the partner different symptomatic, emotional, and mood perceptions [3].

As well as an altered and discontinuous compliance in overcoming both the physical and neurovegetative symptoms, and in the resumption of post-surgical organic functionality, of planning, and of positive perception to the uro-sexological improvement and to the progressive optimization of the quality of life of individuals and of the couple.

Uro-sexual Rehabilitation

- Rehabilitation activities include intervention programs with the patient and the partner
- The research project envisages carrying out rehabilitation activities with the patient and defining support interventions that help him overcome the change (greater sensitivity and emotional lability, psychological impatience, alteration of the perception of enterprise in social, sexual, work, and emotional life)
- Research will focus on the need for rehabilitation and on the different perceptions of the quality of life of the patient and the partner (as individuals and as a couple)

19.7 Before the Prosthesis, Penile Rehabilitation?

Using urologic oncological terminology, "rehabilitation of the penis" is one of the post-surgical phases that contemplates the use of all kinds of surgical interventions (oral and injective intracavernous pharmacological, vacuum erection devices (VED) and any combination of these therapies) in order for the patient to achieve erections suitable for conducting satisfactory sexual intercourse, as well as achieving in the IEFF test an evaluation of the erectile response coefficients equal to the preoperative period.

Clinical experience shows that medication can do much, but the motivation for sexuality also comes from the partner. And from the variables that her biography and clinical history propose:

1. Partners in menopause, with lubrication problems
2. Partners who have undergone cancer surgery for the diagnosis of breast or uterine carcinoma or, for example, for hip replacement, mitral or aortic valvulopathy
3. Partners with a much lower age than the urologic oncological patient (even 10–18 years) in search of a motherhood
4. Partners who, prior to the urologic oncological patient, had lived with partners who were not functioning sexually and were therefore not very cooperative
5. Partners with early menopause (38–39 years old)
6. Partners with sexual dysfunction (excitement disorder, orgasm)
7. Partners with severe depression and deflection of desire
8. Partners with endocrinological syndromes (e.g., Hashimoto syndrome)
9. Homosexual partners, with the characteristics of a sexuality that is far more erotic than heterosexual sexuality
10. Partners with problematic children (character, psychiatric, chronic)
11. Partners with elderly parents to take care of at home
12. Partners who have experienced sexual abuse in childhood or adolescence
13. Partners with serious hormonal pathologies
14. Infertile partners
15. Others

19.8 The Clinical Practice

- *These variables alone, to which many other hypotheses can certainly be added, make penile rehabilitation only a small part of sexual rehabilitation.*
- *Which means:*

- Involving the partner in post-surgical rehabilitation right from the start, 15 days after the hospital discharge.
- Neuro-urologist, neuro-sexologist, and andrologist simultaneously begin to meet the patient and partner.
- Understanding the sexuality of couples.
- Awareness, through the partner of her own gynecological, sexual, and surgical history and her vision of the future.

- Understanding the characteristics of the sexuality of the couple based on their culture of origin, religion, and the experience of individuals.
- With widowed patients, it is possible that occasional partners (former friends, former university partners) and carers can work side by side.

Keep in Mind

Each of these and other variables requires a targeted approach, tailor-made and above all shared with the andrologist responsible for prescribing pharmacological therapies for the rehabilitation of the penis.

In fact, it will not be possible to offer injection therapy to a patient with a phobia of needles or syringes, with religious modesty, with repulsion or reluctance to any means that could be invasive and damaging to his genitality.

19.9 The Therapeutic Process

Encouraging, educating, and motivating couples to regain a quality of life where intimacy can be an important part is an unconscious therapeutic process for the patient and partner.

Both will arrive only at the end of the same process to consider that sexuality is the resumption of a relational, affective, and playful intimacy, inside and outside the bedroom, and not the monotonous repetition of intercourse or of an erectile and orgasmic response, albeit a modified one.

Keep in Mind

It is not without reason that, in order to achieve this goal, the psychosexologist must work to ensure that sexuality loses the feeling of competition with the patient and with an erection that does not always meet expectations. While for the partner, we need to invest in the sensitivity of a woman who shares intimacy, abandoning the roles of nurse and geisha, with a healthy selfishness thinking about herself and her own well-being.

Case 1

"The erection has always been my recurring thought," says Massimo, 58. "After the diagnosis of prostate cancer and the interview, I was afraid of no longer being the same as before...I immediately tried auto-eroticism...and I felt so down...the penis only just lifted up and I was afraid I was changed...then when you gave me the exercises Doctor, ... I felt safe ... I had a guide ... but every time I was alone I tried, whether my penis responded or slept ... It was a long journey but now it's better ... and then you tell me that 'I'd been good' ... and my wife keeps saying that we should have met you earlier doctor ...."

"I do it for Him," says Lucia 58 years. "Sex is not important to me. Since I underwent a hysterectomy (at 47) I have shut down my senses ....The therapies for the hormonal block have done the rest ... the desire has passed ... and when I see him so ardent ... I let him do it ... but doctor, can' t you help my husband without me ... Or at least, don't make me do things ... things ... strange things ...."

A study by Daniela Wittmann et al. [4] examined 20 couples with a biosocial model (analytic induction, with NVivo software), which observed the functional, biological, psychological, and relational aspects of sexuality after radical prostatectomy.

It was found that preoperatively 30% of men reported erectile dysfunction (ED) and 84% of partners were postmenopausal. In addition, the optimism of the surgeon and confidence in the medical team led 90% of couples to overestimate the recovery of erections. The study showed that sexual activity had decreased in frequency and couples reported poor sensitivity (post-traumatic to surgery). In summary, the researchers point out that the sexual recovery of couples requires dealing with sexual function, the sensations of "evisceration" from surgery (removal of the prostate or bladder or a stretch of the colon), and the loss of nerve bundles in those patients where it was not possible to save them from extracapsular cancer (e.g., extra prostate).

Here it is worth emphasizing another point.

19.10 The Charisma of the Surgeon, Urologist, and Andrologist

The style and the personality of the surgeon has a decisive role in making the urologic oncological patient (and the partner) confident of the outcome. The surgeon's most frequent and heartfelt reassurance to the patient, even on the threshold of the operating room, is to save the nerve bundles.

Sometimes, most of the time, this is possible, and other times unfortunately it is not, in order to avoid recurrence in the future.

The fact that the surgeon has done everything possible, in one way or another, makes him "the Prof. par excellence," and the team that will work on rehabilitation, precisely because it was chosen by him, cannot be matched.

Keep in Mind

When the rehabilitation team makes the grade, the patient's disappointment emerges that in that situation of expected excellence, the erection is not the same as before emerges, the feeling of frustration and irascibility of the patient increases disproportionately, incontinence exercises are struggling to give positive results, and learning to change the ostomy, in the case of urinary bypass after cystectomy, makes individuals "different and survivors." But still different from the preoperative.

If the expectations regarding the rehabilitation team are in part disappointed, the patient will increasingly make use of "monitoring visits with Prof… " and will regret having had surgery, comparing himself with friends and acquaintances who, given the same diagnosis, enjoy a better life.

Clinical practice teaches that the charisma of the Prof … must be shared with the patient, limiting the magical expectations of success, although not limiting a quiet euphoria for the success of surgical treatment.

I have learned to teach the patient that POST-TRAUMATIC STRESS requires longer neurological recovery times than physical recovery times. Even though with robotic surgery, the prostatectomized patient is discharged 1 week after the operation, the psychophysical and emotional rehabilitation times take 90–120 days. Divided into the primary rehabilitation process, the stabilizing phase, and the definitive phase where the best quality of life for the patient and the family system is reached.

Take-Home Message

In this time, the patient is always in contact with the Prof…, but every 8–15 days, he meets each of the rehabilitation specialists, and it is with them that he finds himself "the sole protagonist" of the urological, sexual, emotional, relational, social, and working recovery.

19.11 Quality of Life and New Surgical Frontiers

Looking further ahead, radical cystectomy for bladder cancer also implies many changes in body function, with very profound sexual, urinary, and psychological dysfunction.

A study by Hart et al. [5] evaluated the possible psychological benefits associated with a simultaneous urinary derivation and inflatable penile prosthesis. The control group consisted of patients with urinary derivation who had not undergone a penile prosthesis implantation.

The International Literature

The 224 patients participating in the study responded to four different types of questionnaire that explored the different moods, individual sexual history, indices of dissatisfaction with body image, and comfort and discomfort in the new quality of life. In addition to these data, there was also self-reporting by patients regarding physical, psychological, and sexual problems, as well as in the management of the ostomy in urinary derivations. "The bag," as it was called by the majority of patients, caused discomfort in the procedures of hygiene and changing, detriment in sports practices (going to the pool with the bag was for many patients a cause of discomfort and of renunciation of this practice) and in participation in social activities.

Regardless of the type of urinary derivation (ostomy, Kock pouch, ileal conduit), the greatest problems came from sexual and urological functioning. However, those who had also had an inflatable penile prosthesis implanted showed better function (albeit with emotional discomfort caused by changing erectile response) and greater sexual satisfaction.

The timing of penile prosthesis implantation can, therefore, be simultaneous with prostate or bladder urologic oncological surgery, but in most cases the patient will receive this treatment after about a year of attempts at urological improvement (36%) and especially sexual improvement (47%, if before surgery for bladder or prostate cancer or colorectal cancer the patient had a good erectile and orgasmic response and did not complain of dysfunction, unless occasional) [6].

The motivation is not always very strong, and more often it is the last attempt not to feel "too different" especially if the nerve bundles have not been spared.

Keep in Mind

Restoring the elasticity of the tunic and of the vascular cavernous bodies again becomes the priority in the months preceding the prosthetic implantation.

Therapy then with vacuum device (VED device for erection in vacuum) prevents venous-occlusive dysfunction following radical prostatectomy, for example, it preserves the length and circumference of the member [7].

19.12 Penile Prosthesis and the Life of the Couple

Despite all the efforts of surgeons and patients to "bring back to life" individuals who are so tired of disease and post-surgical rehabilitation, some couples, after the implantation of penile prostheses, are dissatisfied with the length of the penis, the circumference, and the swelling of the glans.

A study tried to explore the phenomenon, enlisting 18 couples who had undergone penile prostheses. Only oral PDE5 drugs or intracavernous therapies were administered. The increases, the study claims, were penile circumference of 21% and length of 47.6%. Only one patient was found to have had complications with implant reinsertion.

Take-Home Message

To what extent can the cause of such complaints be psychological? The body image often suffers traumas which are too hard to accept, and the search for sizes and diameters can sometimes be a sort of relentless search, because the diagnosis of cancer, the surgical intervention, and the transformation of the urinary and sexual response had never been accepted.

Case 2

"I sit like a woman …to perform my urinary functions," explains Flavio 61 (prostatectomized). "Standing up has become a memory…not to mention that I always have the fear of leaking a few drops…especially if I laugh for a long time…or worse…I forget to empty my bladder…before sexual intercourse…I am ashamed…I feel defeated…I think that my wife would have every right to leave me…."

More recent studies show high levels of patient and partner satisfaction after penile prosthesis. The research, for example, aimed to evaluate the quality of life, psychological well-being, and satisfaction following prosthetic implantation in patients already surgically treated for prostate cancer.

The Study and Research

Ninety-six patients undergoing prosthetic implantation after RP (radical prostatectomy) and their partners were evaluated between 2010 and 2016. Of this sample, 71 patients and 43 partners individually completed questionnaires on sexual function, psychological well-being, and implant satisfaction, as well as on levels of anxiety and depression. With regard to sexual satisfaction after the implantation of penile prostheses, a comparison was made between male and female satisfaction indices.

Patients filled out the Prostate Cancer Index (EPIC-26), the Index of Erectile Function after Implantation (EDITS), the Quality of Life Scale related to Prostatic Surgery, the Self-Esteem Index, the Questionnaire on Quality of Relationship (SEAR), Generalized Anxiety Disorder (GAD 7), and Patient Health Questionnaire 9 (PHQ9). The partners filled in the questionnaires: GAD 7; PHQ 9; EDITS, Partner Version; and SEAR.

Take-Home Message

Ninety-four percent of patients declared full satisfaction with the treatment of penile prosthesis with good sexual function. Anxiety and depression scores were lower than normal for regained sexual confidence and improved erectile function. Furthermore, patients showed a higher score of sexual satisfaction (90.6%) than their partners, 81.2%.

This may be because the female perception of sexual satisfaction is less linked to the criterion of physiological response and more attentive to the complicity of a couple, to play, to experimentation, and to the harmony (passionate and erotic) of a couple.

19.13 Conclusions

The resumption of sexuality after a prostate, vesical, or colorectal carcinoma is a step-by-step rehabilitation process that requires a strong emotional bond in the couple, a synergistic ability to deal with psychophysical difficulties, and a very deep life motivation. When the surgeon approaches these urologic oncological couples, he observes two individuals who have "survived" a long rehabilitation as well as changes to physical and emotional functionality.

The partners represent an important "therapeutic" presence for the patient who feels accompanied, protected, and understood in the emotional difficulties resulting from the physical and emotional consequences of the surgical removal of vital organs. For the surgical-andrological rehabilitation team, which needs a long-term program that involves the complicity of the emotional and sexual experience of the couple. As if it were a rejuvenated sense of "novelty and lightness" after so much pathology.

Case Illustration

The patient testimonials reveal experiences, feelings, moods, and reflections on life change.

His Words 3

"We started this long affair by chance 16 months ago," says Luigi, 62. "I had accompanied a friend to undergo prostate cancer screening, and out of solidarity I did it myself. Twenty days later, I was in the operating theatre for prostate cancer whilst he (the friend) was serene and happy as always. The operation had made me believe that everything would be easy from there on,...whereas...I did all the pelvic and sexual rehabilitation and in the most beautiful...I did 25 cycles of radiotherapy...After so many upsets, it wasn't enough for me to have saved my skin...Serena (his wife) is only 54...so I became brave and rather than take drug after drug....I chose to have a penile prosthesis...Serena was terrified by this choice of mine...she said that we should not challenge fate...Today I am still doing pelvic exercises for some remaining incontinence,...but at least sexuality is much better... 'If I have to be different' I told myself 'it's better to leak a few drops than to not desire Serena and the other women.'"

His Words 4

"It's two years since I was diagnosed with a superficial bladder tumor and...here I am with the urinary derivation and my 'snack bag' (the ostomy)," says Giovanni Maria, 64. "...I call it that in order to depress myself less...It has been hard to accept this thing (ostomy)....I was ashamed... I was afraid that it would come off ... that I would leak urine ... My friends have always told me that you could not see anything when I was dressed ... and even in my swimming costume ... but I have never believed their opinions completely ... except Franco (a former high school friend) ... He was always loyal. He told me 'sure, you're different...because you don't smile anymore...because you think that nothing is worth it anymore'...It was he, you remember Doctor (psychosexologist) who brought me to you...When you spoke to

me with the surgeon about penile prostheses I said to myself…But what do these two want?…They are quick to speak and to propose…they're healthy! But Franco, who knows me, brought me back to you to speak alone … I remember that you (psychosexologist) told me 'Mr. Giovanni the choice is yours alone. You have to decide whether you want to live as a healthy person or to be a patient for life. Whatever you decide, I will respect that'….When I told Franco, he smiled, and in the following days he asked me 'Have you answered the doctor's question?' … My wife eventually decided … My wife called Franco and they brought me here for the pre-hospitalization … 'now I'm safe, I told myself, everyone wants me to be here' …it's worth living healthily … or at least trying …."

His Words 5

"*My twin sister has been treated for years for Crohn's disease,*" *says Stefano, 46.* "*I thought I was so lucky compared to her, until I had to deal with colon cancer… 'You wanted to even things out at all costs.' was my sister's expression but she (the sister) has always been more tenacious than me….I had just separated and I had been staying for a while with my sister (who is single by choice) … The lawyer … the post-surgical … I couldn't cope … I took antidepressants because my sister insisted so much … desire … sexuality were a long way off. With psychiatric drugs I worked, I played soccer with friends, I spent the weekend with my family. It seemed to me that I had become a grandfather … During a business trip by plane, I talked with the guy in the neighbouring seat… an andrologist surgeon … He understood me immediately … On landing at the airport I asked him for his business card and I thought … 'Maybe one day' … Online, I talked for months every evening with Maria Vittoria and …we saw each other, went out together…and I said that I had to be good enough for this woman…I met you Doctor (psychosexologist) and the surgeon from the plane…and here I am with Maria Vittoria at the first check-up a few weeks after the implantation of penile prosthesis…It's all another life…We live together (with Maria Vittoria)…I feel sorry for my sister who has to undergo another operation….*"

Case Illustration

The partners reveal unusual aspects of the partners and of the couple in a new life experience….

Her Words 1

"*It wasn't easy for Virginio to get used to the neo-bladder (built with a part of the ileum),*" *explains Floriana, 51.* "*Every day he went to the Bank with a bag with a catheter and…everything his …paraphernalia to empty that blessed bladder….Then I was still working part-time to be close to our daughter and I realized that I could not manage to give courage to my husband and care for my daughter … I decided to help myself and for a year I saw a psychotherapist … It has served me so well … and it was there (in therapy) that I discovered that we were young and healthy and with a healthy daughter. We had to live!…I proposed to Virginio he continue the therapy for sexual function but I understood that his motivation was very low…Then, talking with my therapist, he gave me your name….(psychosexologist)…The rest you know …I came with my husband, you listened to us and then you said Mr Virginio would you be kind enough to meet again, alone? If the lady will allow us ... I was very happy that Virginio too had someone to open up with ... Now we have been meeting for two years ... Everything is so different ... Sometimes I think that perhaps it was all a dream ....*"

Her Words 2

"To be frank, foolishly, I envied Carlo," reveals Anna Chiara, 57. "He was followed step by step after the removal of the prostate with a patience that only you therapists have ... When twice they removed nodules from my breast, I was not followed so much ... Sure, the surgeon, the oncologist were very professional. But Carlo had meetings every 15 days and the 'exercises' to do at home...The story of the excercises (pelvic exercises for incontinence and sexual exercises) also made an impression on our children...When they called us on the phone they asked me 'Mum, is dad there? Is he free or is he doing his homework... but above all I didn't feel left out. 'Where is Your Guardian Angel?', you (psychosexologist) asked my husband...and when we told you that we were no longer young, you said 'What do you mean you aren't you young? You're in your second teenage years!' Well, adolescence aside, the penis implant was the natural consequence of seeing Carlo regain motivation and energy. He started sailing again...The implant went well, getting used to this new intimacy...it wasn't easy for me...it seemed so strange to me...but then I could see Carlo was happy...."

Her Words 3

"It's been a really difficult two years," says Elena Lucia, 53. "In one year both of Alessandro's (her husband's) parents died, he underwent surgery for a bladder carcinoma with urinary derivation and ostomy... and finally our first grandson ended up in intensive care immediately after birth. Emotionally collapsing would have been no more than human ... but our daughter needed us ... we had to give her courage for the health of the child ... When we took him home he was really like a wren ... and Alessandro thought that 'if he was going to be a grandfather for a short or a long time... he should get on with it ....' He's done everything himself Alessandro, he changes his ostomy, always travels with an 'emergency kit' (a bag with change of ostomy and cleanser for wound hygiene) and today he is the happiest grandfather in the world ...Luca (his grandson) survived,...he's small...a wren but he's so beautiful...Our daughter works in this Clinic...it was she (her daughter) who told us about you...she told us that we would be...in good hands...."

Patient Guide

What If We Want to Give Some Guidance to the Patient and Partner?

An Example

Hypothesis of disclosures

Guidance for prostatectomized patient and partner

Convalescence and uro-sexual rehabilitation

Dear Patient and Dear Partner,

We would like to provide you with some useful information during your convalescence at home, after your discharge from hospital following radical prostatectomy (removal of the prostate and seminal vesicles).

Below you will find a series of answers to the most common concerns and some suggestions for daily care for a better quality of life.

On the day of discharge, the surgical wound is checked and treated, but it is also important to check the wound at home. Abstaining from hygienic bathing operations until the removal of sutures (which are usually removed after about 10 days from the surgery in the urological outpatient clinic) and from showering until the removal of the bladder catheter.

If the wound appears reddened, hot, and swollen or if serum is leaking from the wound, it is important to consult your urologist surgeon.

After the operation, it seems natural to feel tired, sluggish, and not very resistant to fatigue. However, it is advisable to keep moving at home, avoiding sitting for long and/or lying in bed.

If swelling (edema) appears in the legs, it is advisable to consult the urologist surgeon, while the appearance of edema in the penis and/or scrotum (quite common after a radical prostatectomy operation) often disappears spontaneously after a few days of convalescence.

The appearance of fever after being discharged is often a phenomenon limited to the first few days at home, but if it exceeds 38°, it is advisable to contact the urologist surgeon.

Diet can be liberal (including the assumption of a glass of wine per meal) avoiding, immediately after the operation, particularly substantial foods, rich in fats.

A moderate resumption of physical activity (walking, short domestic errands) improves circulation and breathing. However, it is advisable to resume use of the bicycle and/or mopeds only 8–10 weeks after the operation.

Driving in the car is possible from 2 to 3 weeks after the operation, avoiding long distances. Otherwise, it is advisable to stop every hour and get out of the car to reactivate the circulation of the legs by walking and moving in the parking areas.

Work can be resumed after at least 2–4 weeks of convalescence.

19.14 The Conquest of Autonomy

Urinary continence, resumption of sexual function

Once the catheter is removed, the resumption of continence is the first goal to be reached to gain greater physical autonomy.

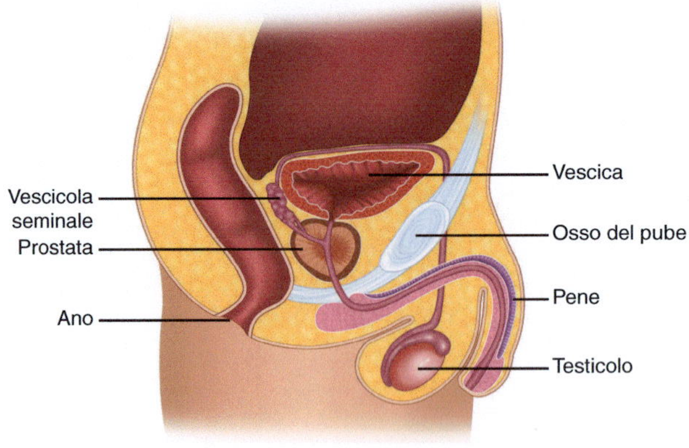

In this phase, the patient's willingness and consistency in conducting specific exercises to strengthen the muscles surrounding the urethra and rectum (pelvic floor), controlling urinary and intestinal function, is important.

Urological rehabilitation involves useful exercises to contract and relax this musculature, facilitating its elasticity when lying down, sitting, or standing. Initially, it may seem difficult to control your muscles and maintain contraction for a long time.

Especially when switching from a sitting position to a standing position, lifting a light weight, coughing, or sneezing suddenly.

During the pelvic floor contraction phase, abdominal, back, buttock, and leg muscles should not be used.

In the initial phase of urological rehabilitation, it may be useful to use biofeedback, a technique by which the patient learns to recognize and contract the pelvic muscles correctly, observing the correct and wrong movements on a computer monitor (connected to an abdominal-perineal or transrectal probe).

As the patient recovers continence, the use of urological aids (diapers and/or pads) to protect the underwear and protect the patient's privacy in public and social contexts is recommended.

The overall recovery time for continence varies from individual to individual, from 2 to 4 months.

19.15 The Therapeutic Role of the Partner

19.15.1 The Resumption of Erectile and Sexual Function

The fear and anxiety of losing one's life to prostate cancer at the time of diagnosis has made surgical intervention a priority, while the resumption of urinary continence after radical prostatectomy too is a priority.

This is accompanied by the thought of being able to verify in the short or medium term the mechanical resumption of erectile function and, immediately afterward, of sexual function.

This natural evolution in the patient's thinking and physical progress does not always coincide with the partner's predisposition to experience the resumption of intimacy as an equally consequent step.

In fact, the male and female approaches to intimacy are different, even before the intervention. As much due to interest as to age, as to previous experiences (sexual, early ejaculation or erectile dysfunction for the patient, orgasm disorder or vaginismus for the partner, and/or oncological, experience of breast or uterine cancer for the partner).

Furthermore, the brain areas connected to sexuality are twice as large in men as in women. Men think, experiment, fantasize, and react to sexuality more frequently than do women. And if they notice a certain reluctance on the part of the partner or only a different frequency of interest and of experimentation, within the couple, of sexual activity, it happens that the men are discouraged, feel less loved, and feel barely liked.

Just like a partner may feel in the case of a decrease in verbal communication, if the man stops talking, he appears more silent and closed, she will think that he is no longer in love or is emotionally distant from her.

In addition to this, there is the surgical technique. Erectile nerves and vessels (vascular-nerve bundles) that make erectile function possible are located close to the prostate.

In some cases, the surgical technique (radical prostatectomy nerve sparing) allows them to be preserved unilaterally or bilaterally, thus reducing the extent of postoperative erectile dysfunction.

In other cases, however, depending on the extent of the tumor, the surgical technique becomes even more radical, and the surgeon must sacrifice not only the prostate but also the erectile nerves.

The absence of erectile function leads the patient into depression, to reduce his quality of life in terms of physical health and to exclude aspects of pleasure.

Sometimes overwhelmed by his partner who, in order to protect the patient, anticipates him, describing the pointlessness of sexual function to doctors, surgeons, and rehabilitation specialists.

While erectile function can be stimulated by appropriate drug therapy (suggested by the urologist surgeon), the spontaneity and naturalness of sexual function can be adequately restored, thanks to the support of the therapeutic role of the partner and by sexological rehabilitation.

Sexological rehabilitation includes space for the patient, the partner, and the couple. This approach, in connection with the urologist surgeon and the urological and pharmacological rehabilitation team, allows, through sexual exercises, the activation of the world of partners' feelings, relationships, and intimacy, recovering male and female relational and sexual desires and needs.

Involving the couple in a rehabilitation process closer to the expectations of the quality of life of the patient and the partner, in harmony with the urologist surgeon.

To further explore the steps of sexual rehabilitation, we include some useful and practical insights:

Characteristics of the Prostate

- The prostate is an organ of the male genital apparatus: it is the size of a chestnut and consists of a muscular part and a glandular part.
- It is located just under the bladder, in front of the rectal intestine (the terminal part of the intestine) and is crossed by a canal called the urethra. The urine and the seminal fluid are released through the latter.
- The main function of the prostate is to produce the prostate secretion (through its glands) which constitutes about 30% of the seminal fluid emitted by the penis during ejaculation.

Prostate and Sexuality
Male sexual response and orgasmic sensation

- The deferent vessels (for the passage of the spermatozoa), the prostate, and the seminal vesicles cause a series of contractions that push the spermatozoa into the urethra
- As soon as these contractions begin, the man feels as if he has reached the limit of control and feels, without being able to stop, the need to ejaculate
- Subsequently, in male orgasm, the contractions of the urethra and penis join those of the prostate and cause ejaculation (the emission of seminal fluid from the tip of the penis)
- The rhythmic contractions of the prostate, the perineum muscles, and the body of the penis (which determine the thrust of the spermatozoa) initially occur at an interval of about 8 s from each other and increase in intensity for the expulsion of the semen during ejaculation
- The sperm will not be ejaculated as it was prior to surgery because of the long journey it has to make through the urethra
- Usually, during ejaculation, the neck of the urinary bladder remains completely closed to allow the passage of sperm (and prevent parts of urine from mixing with the spermatozoa
- Conversely, in patients who have undergone radical prostatectomy, the bladder neck does not close completely during orgasm, and the sperm then flows into the bladder (regressed or retrograde ejaculation)
- To this condition, in patients who have undergone radical prostatectomy, erectile difficulty is added due to the removal of one or both of the nerve bundles that allow erectile function

Orgasm
- This specifically refers to sudden and rhythmic muscle contractions in the pelvic region and other regions of the body that result from a response of the central nervous system (by mental tension, erotic excitement) that accompanies this experience

Ejaculation
- This is the release of sperm and can sometimes occur even in the absence of orgasm. Orgasm without ejaculation is frequent in boys before puberty (adolescence) or in cases of prostate disease, neurological diseases, or drug use

Dedicated to Her

Erectile function, male sensitivity

Precisely because of the different male and female ways of experiencing feelings and passions, including sexual ones, it seems largely difficult for a man to explain to his partner the sense of restlessness and bewilderment, after an intervention of radical prostatectomy.

Even more so the anxiety and disappointment at the partial or total loss of erectile function.

Especially when the patient measures himself by the vulnerability of his body and after the surgical intervention of radical prostatectomy, must measure himself against the loss of one or both bundles of erectile nerves.

The sexual response necessarily changes and loses the spontaneity experienced over the years, and one starts to become familiar with a new way of obtaining an erection and orgasm, now without visible ejaculation (because it is internal, retrograde).

The direct and indirect significance of male upheaval appears to be manifold, as are the reasons for man's dependence on his partner, for a faster recovery of a quality of life appropriate to the individual and his feelings.

Take-Home Message

However, because of differences in physical conformation, sexual response, and emotionality, it is often difficult for a partner to consider this.

Communicating for couples can be made less easy by emotional and relational misunderstandings.

To Her

To facilitate this process, we dedicate to the partner some considerations about the sexual and nonsexual meanings of male erectile function:

- In the erectile act, a man identifies the health of his own body and the strength of his own vitality, that is, "if the body functions, if I obtain an erection like all other men, I feel equal to all other men, I feel like a virile man."
- In the erectile act, a man verifies his capacity to please himself and to please the opposite sex
- With an erection a man can penetrate and enter the body of a woman. He can feel the passionate power of excitement and feel welcomed by his partner.
- Erectile ability allows a man to approach his partner, to embrace her, to kiss her, to feel "worthy" of her passion. To experience passion, exciting thoughts, and feelings.

- The erectile capacity is preparatory to ejaculation, that is, to delivering the seminal liquid into the female body.
- Erectile ability gives pleasure and excitement and produces exciting sensations in the partner. During sexual intercourse, in fact, the apex of the penis (the glans, which contains the final part of the sensory nerves) by stimulating, inside and outside the tissues of the vagina and clitoris, accentuates the threshold of pleasure until orgasm is reached in both partners.

Keep in Mind

The loss of erectile capacity for a partner is mostly experienced as the definitive end of passion, ejaculation, procreation, virility, well-being, strength, security of acquired affections, self-confidence, and the discounted ability to manage events in the outside world. The end of one's own way of being (identity) and acting among others (sexual role).

Affective and relational dependence on the partner inevitably tends to become more accentuated, and *sexual rehabilitation* penetrates and makes complementary the emotional needs of the partner, the virile, and emotional needs of the patient.

On Her Side

Intimacy and feminine sensitivity

- **Why is the erectile act only a sexual response for a woman?**

No specialist, even after the partner's radical prostatectomy intervention, appears accustomed to asking the partner "How do you feel? What are you going through?"

Talking to women about intimacy, erectile function, and rehabilitation of male post-surgical sexology may seem like distant requests that are alien to their emotions at the time.

Analogously, identifying in a man's erectile act, and in his claim, any other meaning than sexual. Especially if the partner still seems to be afraid of cancer diagnosis and surgery.

Take-Home Message

The sexological rehabilitation service also foresees, with the help of the specialist sexologist, the clarification with the partner of doubts and disorienting sensations in this regard, using as an analogy, for example, the process of sexual rehabilitation of the partner, with what a woman would experience after an operation of removal of the uterus and ovaries (hysterectomy).

She would more easily understand the changed relationship with her body, her femininity, and the way she was a woman, wife, mother, and friend, before the surgery. She would feel anguished by the fear of losing her partner's love, of not being a seductive woman for him, and of not being able to be the woman of before.

Keep in Mind

Not forgetting the verbal, affective, and sexual communication of the couple.

The patient and the partner have experienced, each within himself/herself, the fear of seeing truncated (because of neoplasia and/or surgical consequences), the project of life for two. They have thought a lot between the time of diagnosis and the surgical intervention.

Today, they feel the need to be reassured and to come together again.

In communication, in affection, in relationships, and in intimacy.

In this sense, post-surgical sexological rehabilitation aims to facilitate the patient and the partner in a "second project of the man and a second project of the couple", by preparing individual rehabilitation protocols (for the patient and for the couple) together with the urologist specialist.

Dear patient and partner, we would like to thank you for your kind attention and would like to be able to accompany you in your sexual rehabilitation, in order to achieve a better quality of life for you.

19.16 Self-Check Path

We would just like to verify our therapeutic style and the characteristics of our therapeutic contract with the patient.

1. A 52-year-old widower with a mitral valvulopathy asks for a consultation for a penile prosthesis implant: your first thought is to contact the heart surgeon, ask the patient the reasons for this request, and evaluate with the patient the expectations of success of the implant.
2. When in the interview with the patient, you realize that the partner is against the prosthetic implant: you try to understand the reasons, you think that the partner is an obstacle to be sent to the psychosexologist, and you propose a further meeting in the presence of the psychosexologist.
3. Contraindications of a prosthetic implant: leave you indifferent, you think they are part of the surgical routine, and you worry about the clinical solution to be provided and the patient's reaction.
4. The request for a penile prosthesis after radical cystectomy: it seems a reasonable choice to you, you try to examine how the patient came to this hypothesis,

and you make sure that the patient's motivation does not hide depressive or psychiatric syndromes.
5. Give antidepressant drugs to patients stressed by post-prostatectomy incontinence: this seems to be a healthy precaution, you do not think the prescription is useful, and you make sure that the patient has experienced post-traumatic stress.
6. The post-traumatic surgical stress to a colon cancer seems to you a normal neurovegetative reaction that does not require any kind of vigilance, is the subject of the psychosexologist, and is a topic that does not interest surgeons.
7. A patient with urinary derivation and neo-bladder ileal is for you a very complex patient, a case of undoubted interest, and a difficult patient.
8. The psychosexologist can be for a surgeon a colleague who does not create a problem, a colleague of secondary importance, and a colleague who can resolve difficult situations.

19.17 Medical History Questions

19.17.1 For the Patient

1. How did you come to the hypothesis of a penile prosthesis implant?
2. What has suffered most from rehabilitation after radical prostatectomy?
3. How can penile prosthesis implantation, beyond offering you better erectile function, help improve your future?
4. How important is sexuality to you?
5. Have you had sexual dysfunction in your previous relationships?
6. How are you experiencing the new orgasm with retrograde ejaculation?
7. Is your partner a sexual partner?
8. How has your life changed since after cancer diagnosis and surgical treatment?
9. Have you had radiotherapy after radical prostatectomy?
10. Which therapies have given the best results for sexual function, after radical cystectomy?
11. What kind of outcome do you expect from a penile prosthesis implantation?

19.17.2 For the Partner

1. How does your partner seem today? Does he seem tired by his experience of prostate cancer?
2. How did you feel during all these months of urological and sexual rehabilitation?
3. How did you both come to think of a new surgical implant?
4. What frightens you most about the situation?
5. Do you think your partner has sufficient emotional resources to overcome this new surgery?

6. How important has sexuality been in your relationship so far?
7. Which of you is more attentive to intimacy?
8. Have you also had surgery? What for?
9. From the gynecological point of view, have you faced any particular pathologies?
10. Have you ever thought that penile prostheses could make your partner more sexually extroverted and eager for other experiences?
11. What do you fear most for yourself? And what do you hope to be positive for yourself in this situation?

References

1. Billings D, Folkman S, Acree M, Moskowitz J (2000) Coping and physical health during caregiving: the roles of positive and negative effect. J Pers Soc Psychol 79:131–142
2. Golden Kreutz D, Thornton L, Wells DiGregorio S, Frierson G, Jim H, Karpenter K, Shelby R, Andersen B (2005) Traumatic stress, perceived global stress and life events: prospectively predicting quality of life in breast cancer patients. Health Psychol 24:288–296
3. Delongis A, Holtzman S (2005) Coping in context: the role of stress, social support, and personality in coping. *J Pers* 73:1633–1656
4. Wittmann D et al (2015) What the couple on recovery of sexual intimacy after prostatectomy: towards the development of a conceptual model of sexual couple recovery after surgery for prostate cancer. J Sex Med 12(2):494–504
5. Hart S et al (1999) Quality of life after radical cystectomy for bladder cancer in patients with an ileal conduit, bag of skin or urethral Koch. J Urol 162(1):77–81
6. Tsikis ST et al (2017) The relationship between incontinence and erectile dysfunction after robotic prostatectomy: mutually exclusive? J Sex Med 14(10):1241–1247
7. Pahlajani G et al (2012) Vacuum erection devices, showing: the emerging role in the treatment of erectile dysfunction and early rehabilitation of the penis after prostate cancer therapy. J Sex Med 9(4):1162–1189

Bibliography

Di Matteo M, Giordani PJ, Lpper HS, Croghan TW (2002) Patient adherence and medical treatment outcomes: a meta-analysis. Med Care 40:794–811

Dunmore E, Clark DM, Ehlers A (2001) A prospective investigation of the role of cognitive factors in persistent post-traumatic stress disorder (PTSD) after physical or sexual assault. Behav Res Ther 39:1063–1084

Epstein RM (2004) Patient trust: is it related to patient-centred behaviour of primary care physicians? Med Care 42:1049–1055

Fredriksson M et al (1989) Colon cancer, physical activity, and occupational exposures. A case-control study. Cancer 63:1838–1842

French D, Maissi E, Marteau T (2005) The purpose of attributing cause: beliefs about the causes of myocardial infarction. Soc Sci Med 60:1411–1421

Haley W, Lamonde L, Han B, Burton A, Schonwetter R (2003) Predictors of depression and life satisfaction among spousal caregivers in hospice: application of a stress process model. J Palliat Med 6:215–224

Mac Keown-Eyssen G (1994) Epidemiology of colorectal cancer revisited: triglycerides in serum and/or plasma glucose associated risk. Cancer Epidemiol Biomarkers Prev 3:687–695

O'Connor R (2005) Undoing perpetual stress: the missing connection between depression, anxiety, and 21st century illness. Berkley, New York

Pakenham K (2001) Application of a stress and coping model to caregiving in multiple sclerosis. Psychol Health Med 6:13–27

Peralta-Ramirez M, Jimenez-Alonso J, Godoy-Garcia J, Perez-Garcia M (2004) The effects of daily stress and stressful life events on the clinical symptomatology of patients with lupus erythematosus. *Psychosom Med* 66:788–794

Akin-Olugbade O, Parker M, Guhring P et al (2006) Determinants of patient satisfaction following penile prosthesis surgery. J Sex Med 3:743–748

Chartier-Kastler E, Amar E, Chevallier D et al (2008) Does management of erectile dysfunction after radical prostatectomy meet patients' expectations? Results of a national survey (REPAIR) by the French Urological Association. J Sex Med 5:693–704

Gontero P, Fontana F, Zitella A et al (2005) A prospective evaluation of efficacy and compliance with a multistep treatment approach for erectile dysfunction in patients after non-nerve sparing radical prostatectomy. BJU Int 95:359–365

Hollenbeck BK, Dunn RL, Wei JT, Montie JE et al (2003) Determinants of long-term sexual health outcome after radical prostatectomy measured by a validated instrument. J Urol 169:1453–1457

McCullough AR (2001) Prevention and management of erectile dysfunction following radical prostatectomy. Urol Clin North Am 28:613–627

Mulhall JP, Bella AJ, Briganti A et al (2010) Erectile function rehabilitation in the radical prostatectomy patient. J Sex Med 7:1687–1698

Salonia A, Castagna G, Capogrosso P, Castiglione F, Briganti A, Montorsi F (2014) Prevention and management of post prostatectomy erectile dysfunction. Transl Androl Urol 4(4):421–437. https://doi.org/10.3978/j.issn.2223-4683.2013.09.10

Tal R, Alphs HH, Krebs P, Nelson CJ et al (2009) Erectile function recovery rate after radical prostatectomy: a metaanalysis. J Sex Med 6:2538–2546

Tal R, Lindsay M, Jacks MS et al (2011) Penile implant utilization following treatment for prostate cancer: analysis of the SEER-Medicare database. J Sex Med 8:1797–1804

Penile Prosthesis Implant for Severe Erectile Dysfunction

20

Elena Vittoria Longhi and Fulvio Colombo

20.1 Introduction

Male erectile dysfunction has multifactorial characteristics that involve an alteration in any one of the components of the response itself: organic, relational, and psychological. Endocrine, neurogenetic, vasculogenic, and iatrogenic causes, metabolic syndromes, and cardiovascular diseases are considered in the evaluation of the diagnosis.

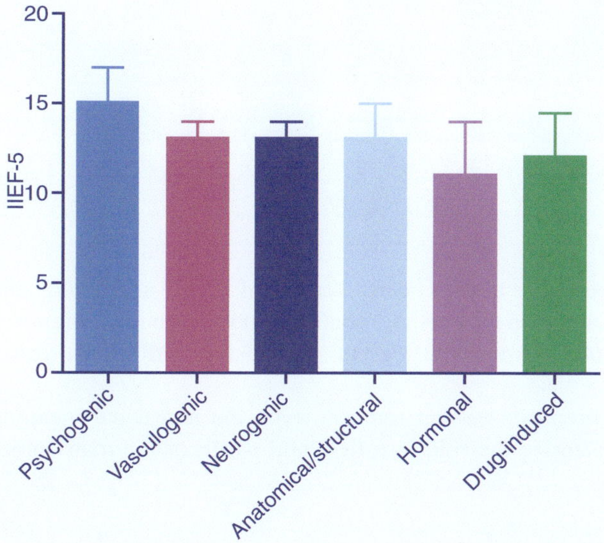

E. V. Longhi et al., *Psychosexual Counseling in Andrological Surgery*,
https://doi.org/10.1007/978-3-319-99646-2_20

Initially, minimally invasive therapies are prescribed to alleviate the symptoms of erectile dysfunction, such as oral drugs, injected vasodilators, and vacuum device.

Normally, surgical therapies, such as penile prosthesis implantation, are reserved for patients presenting adverse pharmacotherapy effects, who complain of penile fibrosis or vascular penile insufficiency.

- IIEF-5 scores of 3151 patients with different pathophysiological causes. Error bar: interquartile range. Kruskal-Wallis H tests for all groups, all organic groups (except for psychogens): P = 0,000 and P = 0,073, respectively
- The severity of ED is increased with age. Spearman's correlations for 3151 patients: rs = −0,198, P = 0,000.

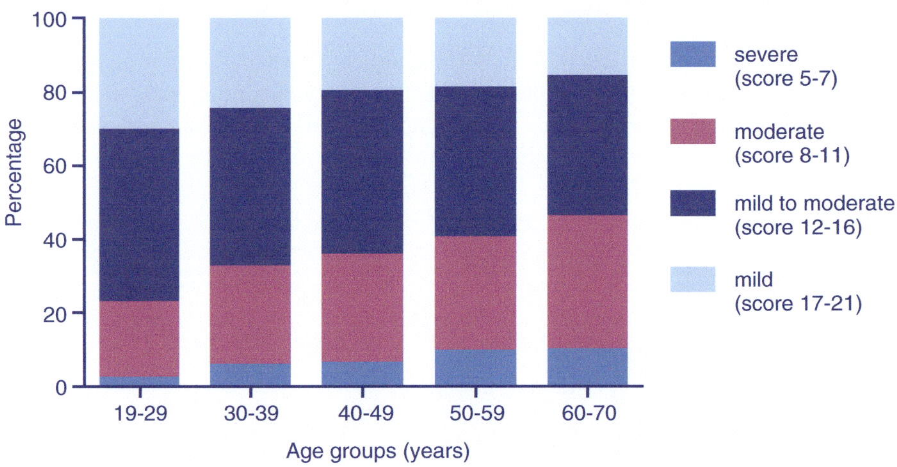

The erect penis has always been a symbol of virility and sexual ability, but it has also been synonymous with social "control," "power" in the professional world, and "affective virtue" toward the partner: "since they are virile, you deserve your affections."

From this premise, we can see how even the nonsexual meanings of erectile function characterize the role, prestige, and worth of the man among men in the world.

Keep in Mind

In the clinical world, the severity of erectile dysfunction is described as LIGHT, MODERATE, OR **SEVERE**, according to the questionnaire of the Index of Erectile Function (IIEF) in five bands: from 1–7 SEVERE, 8–11 MODERATE, 12–16 LIGHT-MODERATE, 17–21 LIGHT, and 22–25 good erectile performance.

It is important to note that erectile dysfunction is no longer simply limited to sexual activity, but also acts as an indicator of systemic endothelial dysfunction [1] or as a sentinel symptom of cardiovascular events or major cardiovascular diseases [2].

Make a Note

And again, alcohol and smoking have been shown to have a significant impact on erectile function [3, 4], as have diets poor in whole foods, legumes, vegetables, fruits, fatty red meat, whole milk products, sweetened foods, and drinks [5].

Metabolic syndromes and obesity are further risk factors affecting erectile function, as are type 1 and type 2 diabetes and also a prediabetic condition [6–8].

Predisposing factors aside, patients with severe erectile dysfunction (refractory to medical therapy or suffering from penile fibrosis secondary to Peyronie's disease, prolonged priapism or serious infections, structural and/or vascular penile defects due to genital or pelvic trauma) are candidates for the implantation of penile prostheses.

Depending on the underlying pathology, the andrologist surgeon will choose one of the most suitable devices for the treatment of erectile dysfunction.

20.2 The Andrological Approach

The primary goal of the penile prosthetic surgery is to allow the patient to recover penetrative sexual activity.

In the last decades, the use of penile prosthesis has become the gold standard therapy for medically refractory ED.

For a long time, penile prosthesis (PP) implants have been considered as the third-line therapy, to be reserved for patients not responsive to other less invasive treatments such as phosphodiesterase-5 inhibitors, intraurethral administrations or intracavernosal injections, and vacuum erection devices.

Nowadays this traditional view should be reconsidered, since prosthesis implant could be proposed as the best option even at the beginning of treatment, depending on the specific needs of the patient. Obviously, the accurate patient selection is of primary importance in PP surgery, in order to reduce risk for postoperative dissatisfaction. For the same reasons, an appropriate and thorough informed consent is a pivotal aspect in the doctor-patient relationship, since the patient's postoperative satisfaction is always related to his preoperative expectations.

Take-Home Message

During nearly 50 years of experience in this surgery, many different contributions have been proposed to establish the correct surgical steps, prevent infection, and manage possible intraoperative and postoperative complications. The continuing enhancements in the quality of employed materials have greatly improved the overall satisfaction, among the operated patients, with significantly lower complication rates.

The updated models of inflatable prosthesis allow the patient to achieve a condition of perfect erection, and, at the same time, they guarantee a natural aspect of complete flaccidity of the penis.

In particular:

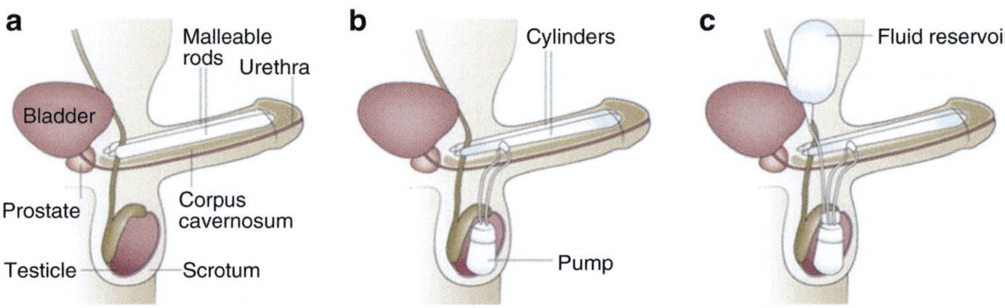

Penile Prostheses: The Types

(**a**) The malleable penile prosthesis involves two semirigid bars that are placed in the corpora cavernosa. The implant changes size; it is bent upward before sexual intercourse. (**b**) The two-piece inflatable penile prosthesis (IPP) involves the placement of two inflatable cylinders in the corpora cavernosa and a pump in the scrotum. When the pump is used, fluid is transferred between the pump and cylinders. (**c**) The three-piece IPP involves positioning two inflatable cylinders (in the corpora cavernosa), a pump in the scrotum and a liquid reservoir in the lower abdomen next to the bladder. The pressure applied to the pump causes a transfer of fluid from the reservoir to the cylinders, resulting in stiffness of the penis. The pump has a release valve or button to transfer fluid from the cylinders to the reservoir at the end of sexual intercourse.

Thus, these devices permit an excellent concealment when deactivated, reducing risk of erosion and allowing normal urethral instrumentation, when required.

The informed consent should clearly describe the advantages and disadvantages of the procedure, other treatment options, limitations, and possible complications such as infection and its consequences; bleeding; pain; mechanical failure; penile shortening; change in sensation and shape; injury to local structures including the urethra, bladder, bowel, or vessels; and autoinflation.

20.3 The Surgical Technique

The operative decision to place a malleable, two-piece, or three-piece IPP is based on several factors, including patient preference, surgeon experience, indication for procedure, manual dexterity, penile size, and mental function. Malleable devices require less manual dexterity by the patient and can be performed under local anesthesia. Given the nature of malleable devices, they are less prone to malfunction; however, they are permanently firm and have lower overall satisfaction compared with three-piece devices.

Keep in Mind

Two-piece IPPs (inflatable penile prosthesis) do not require placement of a separate reservoir and therefore can be used in cases in which reservoir placement is problematic, such as after major pelvic surgery or renal transplantation. With the lack of a distinct reservoir, the two-piece devices do not permit complete deflation of the penile cylinders.

The most common device implanted in penile surgery is the three-piece IPP. The overall proportion of IPP compared with malleable prosthesis increased from 2.3:1 in 2003 to 25:1 in 2012.

The availability of smaller diameter models permits easier placement in cases of significant corporal scarring or decreased tunic elasticity.

Patients are instructed at discharge from the hospital to wear supportive underwear for the first month and direct their penis upward if possible. Patients are taught how to operate their hydraulic devices approximately 4–6 weeks after surgery. Some surgeons prefer to begin cycling devices sooner, but in most patients, pain will be a limiting factor to early cycling. After patients are instructed in the operation of their device, they are advised to cycle regularly.

20.4 The Literature and Clinical Practice

Numerous studies have reported high satisfaction rates for patients and their partners after PP implantation for the treatment of ED (98% patient and 96% partner satisfaction rates).

One of the most common complaints in men receiving a PP is that there is subjective and objective loss of penile length owing to scarring, fibrosis, and general loss of elasticity from altered tissues qualities.

Frequently, patients compare their current with their previous appearance when they had a fully functional erection. This issue and unrealistic expectations and body changes such as weight gain and excess pubis fat can lead a frustrating perception. It is important that the physician discuss these issues with the patient and take a preoperative stretched flaccid penis length measurement for postoperative comparison.

One proposal has been to use physical therapy, in the form of a vacuum or traction device, before implantation to stretch the tissue as much as possible to implant a larger device.

20.5 The Sexual Approach

20.5.1 Through It All, What Are the Feelings of the Patient?

Whatever the chosen device, there is no doubt that erectile dysfunction, having deleterious effects on a man's quality of life, induces the patient to prolonged states of:

1. Anxiety
2. Depression
3. Anhedonia (absence of pleasure)
4. Frustration
5. Physical, emotional, and social inadequacy
6. Loss of the partner due to lack of adequate sexual performance
7. Social phobia
8. Irritability, impatience, and aggression in social and family relations
9. Lack of motivation in every field: family, work, sporting, social, etc.
10. Emotional shutdown, emotional distancing from the partner
11. Abstinence from sexual relations (lack of initiative)
12. Skepticism of and frustration toward the resolution of sexual problem
13. Panic attacks in stressful extra sexual situations

If we consider that the percentage of men, between 40 and 70 years of age, who complain of erectile dysfunction and depression reaches up to 50%, we can guess the altered psychic state with which patients apply for the treatment of penile prosthesis implant. Studies carried out in the United States, Finland, Brazil, Japan, and Malaysia bear witness to this [9, 10].

Given the psychological consequences of erectile dysfunction, it is not surprising that many men have difficulty accepting their condition and avoid any kind of treatment.

Clinical research indicates that 69% of patients deny the existence of erectile dysfunction and the average time to access a first specialist examination is more than 2 years, from the onset of the disorder.

In the Latin world and in particular in Italy, it is often the partners who encourage the patients to face the problem, and, thanks to their insistence, men arrive at a diagnosis and a treatment, initially with skepticism, then depending on the progress, with a regained self-confidence.

Case 1

"They even sent me to talk to a psychologist" says Fabio, 45, "but I wasn't convinced and I let it lie. I asked myself: 'why do they say it's a head problem in addition to hypertension?...so when Dr. ... proposed a consultation with you (Psycho-sexologist) ... I didn't want to come ... then Clara (his wife) threatened me 'either you get better or I divorce you' ... and I realized that she was serious and now I feel more confident ..." "We could have come sooner" reiterates Clara (his wife) "if it hadn't been for me...he has no fantasy...you don't touch it all day...there is only sexual intercourse (...less and less frequent...), his anxiety about the erection and I...don't exist...intimacy is all about seeing if the sexual function is good ... and every time it fails ... he sůlks, does not speak, goes out alone with the dog ... and you can't touch him.... Doctor if you knew how much I have suffered in recent years ...."

Patients generally report experiencing deep disappointment and shame in the face of yet another erectile dysfunction, and even when they use pharmacological treatments, they remain afraid of failure and are inclined to avoid all situations that might lead to a moment of intimacy and sexual intercourse.

Clinical research indicates that 50–80% of men stop using medical and pharmacological treatments for erectile dysfunction within 1 year [11, 12], while discontinuance of the inhibitory use of PDE5 is estimated at 30–50%.

The lack of therapeutic continuity leads to further anguish, anxiety, and relational difficulties. Why?

Case 2

"It's the head that doesn't work because I'm stubborn," says Alessio, 38. "When I see Veronica (his girlfriend; they can only see each other at weekends because they live in different cities), I say to myself 'You only have two days, the weekend, you have to have more sexual intercourse because you are more likely to succeed.' ...then nothing...sometimes, even taking the drug (for impotence) nothing happens...then I say to myself 'See? You're sick. You have to try again and again, otherwise you will never succeed'...You have to do it...."

Besides, not even:

20.6 The Strike of Lysistrata

20.6.1 What Are the Feelings of the Partner?

The partners of men with erectile dysfunction are not immune to frustration, anxiety, anger, and feelings of inadequacy as they address the patient's sexual problem.

The more resistant he is to each kind of treatment, the more disappointed and anxious the partner is.

In fact, partners report disengagement of mood and libido because he drags them into an "early old age" and into a state of absolute denial of health, pleasure, and playing for the couple.

Case 3

"How many times have I suggested to him that we just take a shower together," says Paola, 49, "only to hear the answer 'I prefer to take a shower alone…in the bathroom I want to be alone with my thoughts….' 'But it's fun!' I replied… and he answered 'the time for fun and games is long gone, you are an adult…' In those moments I hated him with all my might … Why couldn't he understand that I was helping him?"

In the two-way dynamics of frustration, deprivation, anger, and depression, misunderstandings increase at every turn, and if the partner demands pleasure for herself and for her own feminine health, the patient with erectile dysfunction feels guilty because he is depriving the partner of all kinds of pleasure.

Take-Home Message

Clinical research on the sexual function of partners of patients with erectile dysfunction (using the FSFI questionnaire) has also shown that women experience hypoactive sexual desire, lack of excitement, and low intensity orgasm (with autoeroticism) [13].

As always, sexual dysfunction is not only a problem for the single individual but also for the couple and is very often underestimated.

In fact, the success of pharmacological and/or surgical treatments depends largely on the type of couple and the basic bond between the partners and the style of the couple: confrontational, symbiotic, aggressive, passive, etc.

Keep in Mind

Confrontational couples will tend to experience the intervention of the drug and/or surgery as a third element of competition and power ("let's see who has more power in the couple."). Symbiotic couples will experience the therapeutic decision in a sense of "all or none," where if only one of the partners were not in agreement, he/she would feel a great sense of guilt. Couples with an aggressive communicative style will put themselves in a "defensive" position toward the treatments (they will argue with the specialist about every side effect and report hypochondriac symptoms). Passive couples will experience every therapeutic intervention without any complaint.

These are just a few variations among the communicative styles of couples.

This leads to reflection: unlike the clinical hypothesis, medication, like the penile prosthetic implant, is experienced by the couple also as an element which conditions the communication between the two.

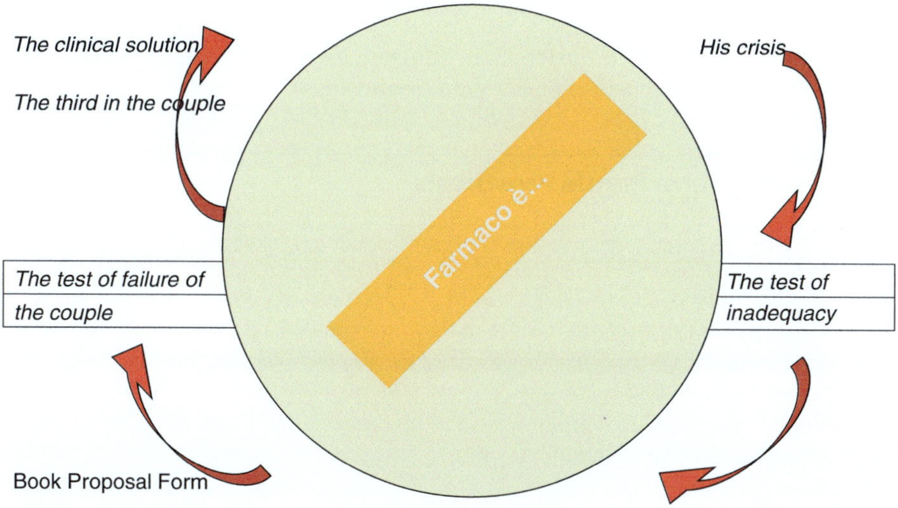

20.7 The International Studies

Not by chance:

A further study by Fisher et al. [14] interviewed 293 partners of patients with erectile dysfunction, via email and using online questionnaires. Patients underwent pharmacological treatment with PDE5 inhibitors. In this research too, the decrease in female sexual satisfaction prior to the partner taking the drug therapy emerged.

Take-Home Message

However, clinical experience, at least in Italy, shows the partner's aversion to the prolonged use of powerful drugs that can undermine the impact of female seductiveness on the patient's erectile response.

Almost as if to say: "If the drug nullifies my feminine allure… you can have erections without me and … so… I'm worth nothing…."

Let us not forget that even the partners of patients with erectile dysfunction may report problems with excitement, orgasm, and desire.

The study by Jiann et al. [13] evaluated female sexual function and erectile function with self-evaluation questionnaires: FSFI (Female Sexual Index) and IIEF (International Index for Erectile Function).

Here, 632 sexually active couples participated in the research, with an average age of 36.9 for women and 39.5 for men.

According to the FSFI and IIEF scores, 42.9% of women reported sexual difficulties, and 15% of men reported erectile dysfunction.

This leads to the hypothesis that men's erectile dysfunction could be a condition of sexual malaise for the partners, but also the partners themselves could be concealing, behind HIS erectile dysfunction, difficulties with excitation, orgasm, sexual satisfaction, and sexual pain at penetration (vaginismus).

20.8 Long-Term Penile Prosthesis

- *Achieving the goal of penile prosthesis implantation is therefore a real clinical journey for the patient and the partner, understood as a step-by-step process of anamnesis, observation, and review of the sexuality of the couple* by the andrologist surgeon and the psycho-sexologist.
- Scientific studies support this practice with positive long-term implant outcomes and with a couple satisfaction ranging from 75 to 100% [15] depending on the prosthetic device.

Having said that, the system foresees a preparatory period with the vacuum pump, 5–10 min, every day, to improve the internal vasodilation and the elasticity of the external tunic, on a mechanical level. The use of andrological exercises for the penis becomes associated with an intensification of the neurological area of excitation, prescribing to the patient the association of erotic fantasies to the use of the vacuum device.

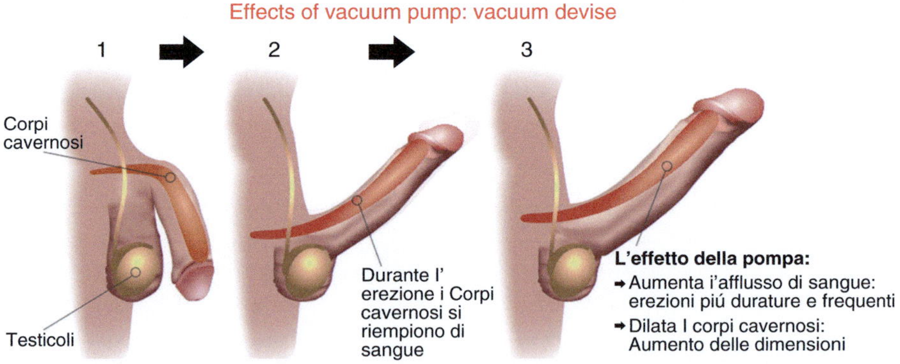

On the other hand, the use of films or visual pornographic material, during operation with the vacuum pump, induces in the patient a greater psychological passivity that will further aggravate the feelings of frustration and resignation of the man who chooses a "prosthetic implant to rekindle his virility."

These exercises should be repeated also in the period following the implantation, alternating between expansion and reduction sequences of the prosthesis for a better adaptation of the same.

Keep in Mind

The partners, from a practical point of view, are very complicit in this further step: "gymnastics," as they often call it, does not interfere with femininity, seduction, passion, and pleasure.

They act as a sort of "personal trainer" for the partner and then moving on, in the sexual act, to "try" the functionality of the implant, with a disclaimer. Almost to say "now that He "works" I can just think of myself and enjoy the pleasure."

If, on the other hand, the partner had shown sexual dysfunctions during her sexual history, during his preparatory phase (with vacuum device), she would be involved with individualized "sexological exercises" according to the disorder of desire, excitement, orgasm, or pelvic pain.

The penile prosthesis implant, seen from this point of view, could also act as a catalyst for the motivation of the couple to overcome sexual difficulties, both individual and of the couple, with a renewed will.

He puts behind him, the long process of suffering and vain previous attempts, to think only of "the here and now" and "the fruits of tomorrow."

20.9 Conclusions

Bioengineering offers surgeons various types of penile prostheses with different surgical implications for different implants, which are increasingly amenable to the needs of the patient and to the individuals' clinical history.

Take-Home Message

However, when implanting a prosthesis, it is vital *to understand "who" the implant is for, "what sexual experience the patient intends," "at what moment in life he decided on this treatment" (after a heart attack, a radical prostatectomy, after a diagnosis of diabetes, etc.), and "what kind of relationship the couple has" (recent, in crisis, long shared). And finally, what role can the partner play, depending not only on her personal clinical history but also on her character (combative, passive, gregarious, etc. and hence her compliance)?*

In all of this, the psycho-sexologist can become a silent director of the dynamics between the couple and the medical team, a facilitator of clinical process for both parties, and a "Jiminy Cricket" who emphasizes the most important aspects of the couple or the medical team to avoid conflicts, misunderstandings, and dissatisfaction.

Case Illustration

His Voice 1

"It's two years that I've had my penile prosthesis," says Flavio, 51. "I had four stents (cardiologic) 5 years ago, and then, the emergency doctor told me 'Be thankful that today is Friday 17th…it has brought you luck and your neck has been saved…' 'I don't know how many Friday 17ths there are in the year, but every time one comes around I go out with my friends for dinner until late….' Then, not having a steady girlfriend (I lived with someone 11 years, it ended in a betrayal … mine) for some time, sexuality has been very random and mostly brought about through my work, for which I travel … But that Friday 17th changed my life….I feel older, more tired, with less energy. My best friend convinced me to have a penile prosthesis…because I was increasingly having less sexual intercourse and leaving my potency drugs at home…during my travels. I am less depressed now, I know I have a 'prosthesis for a friend' … but now I would like a real relationship … who knows if a woman would accept a 'bionic husband' …."

His Voice 2

"I've always been a quick and rational type," says William 61. "I'm an organicist and at my grand old age I was beaten by feelings. I have always solved everything with therapies and surgical treatments: gallstones, reflux therapy, hypertension therapy, alphalythics for prostate hypertrophy… But after retirement… my rationality went walkabout… My wife Sofia had surgery for malignant breast cancer and also had cycles of chemotherapy… I felt lost…I seemed to have lost all hope … I was very close to Sofia and I admired her for the determination and will to get better … After a year of transition, my wife told me 'I'm too young to live an early old age' … Seeing my erectile difficulties … and the poor efficacy of the drugs … we opted for a penile prosthesis and as you know, doctor (psycho-sexologist), everything is just like before. Sexuality came back spontaneously and naturally… but my fear of losing Sofia never left me… and I can't deny that I felt 'saved' when you (psycho-sexologist) asked me 'How many other half-truths do you have to tell yourself before you accept that you are afraid of being alone'… Bullseye! That was my wife's comment and…the rest you know…for the first time I admitted that 'human beings bring people together'…even a stranger can…."

His Voice 3

"To feel rejuvenated at 46 seems like a nonsense," says Alfio, "but for me it was like that…I've always lived in a family of women: my mother, three sisters, an aunt (maternal) and my father and I. I was the second and my sister Vanessa, the first-born, is a battering ram. Very good at studying, very good at work, very good at sport, …I was just the opposite … when I fell in love I thought I knew everything about women … whereas in fact, sex was a fiasco…. For eight years I had panic attacks, depression, cyclothymia, …the medication for mood swings affected my sexual performance…I lost many partners for this reason…until I met a former high school friend…Matilde… a urologist and an andrologist! 'What a relief,' I said to myself 'I can feel at home'…She immediately took me to see a colleague and a month later I was 'brand new'…with a 'life-saving prosthesis…' The trouble is…that I fell in love with my former classmate….

Case Illustration

Her Voice 1

"When I met William he was a young man full of life, he made me laugh and sexuality was spontaneous, natural, fulfilling," says Sara, 39. "Two years of engagement and one year of marriage today. William has changed a lot…six months ago his twin brother died in a car accident and William stopped going out with his friends and wanting sex …he threw himself into work…I even feared he wanted to end the marriage…but he constantly pleads 'Please make sure you'll always be with me.'…Despite the fact that reassuring him is useless … We are here with you Doctor (psycho-sexologist), prosthesis aside, because William has suffered from psoriasis for a month, even on his genitals, it's a nightmare." "Sorry if I went before you" (addresses William during the interview), but the doctor hasn't examined you and would not have known … "do you want me to leave you alone with her (psycho-sexologist) …?"

Her Voice 2

"Rodolfo is my second husband," says Flavia, 61. "My first husband betrayed me continuously and I left him. To now have a man with erectile difficulties at my side,… at the beginning, I am ashamed to say, this reassured me, 'He won't make me suffer' I selfishly told myself. But the situation didn't improve. First, the family doctor prescribed him a drug for potency…the first three times it went well…then 'cold water'…and he became increasingly depressed. Then they gave him drugs to inject and the andrologist said to me 'Help your husband.' And with my history as a nurse, it was I who gave him the injections. Too bad I couldn't detach my mind and behave like a lover… I approached the doctors where I worked and they suggested this department. … Ironically, it was I who convinced Rodolfo to have a penile prosthesis… I can't deny that now I am really afraid that he will betray me too… If he becomes potent again… he will be desirable again, too desirable."

Her Voice 3

"Sexuality has always been a problem for me…" says Alessia, 42. "I haven't had many partners and I don't have much experience…with Claudio (her husband) it was difficult right away. I have suffered from vaginismus since my first sexual intercourse at 19…and I have never got rid of it…my gynecologist says that 'it's a head problem' but going into analysis for years, the thought depresses me. We chose not to have children … but Claudio insisted that I should live peacefully, including sexually. I tried with localized therapies, creams, gels …the pain is always there, … sometimes more bearable, sometimes less … then Claudio discovered that he had diabetes, like all his family on his father's side, and from then on … the situation has become devastating. At each encounter he was tense and focused only on his erectile function….After months of discussions and quarrels, we said that before thinking about a separation, we had to do something…We came to this facility for a penile prostheses implant and to solve my problem…maybe together we can do it…."

20.10 Self-Check Path

There are no right or wrong answers. This is just a way to compare ourselves with our clinical practice and our therapeutic style, without criticism or judgment.

1. When a widower asks you for a penile prosthesis implant, what are your concerns? What do you need to know?
2. How much do you know about the sexual history of the patient's partner?
3. If there is no psycho-sexologist in your department, to whom do you entrust the couple's sexual history?
4. Do you think that a psychiatrist has the same skills as a psycho-sexologist?
5. If you could ask the psycho-sexologist to take care of a part of your difficult anamnesis, which part would you entrust to him?
6. What do you think you have learned from the follow-ups with the patients to whom you have given a penile prosthesis?
7. If you experience a serious complication after a penile prosthesis implant, what are you concerned with initially?
8. How much do you think your personal charisma contributes to the contract with this particular type of patient?
9. How do you assess patient and partner satisfaction? Only within erectile parameters?
10. If a homosexual patient challenges you about a prosthetic implant or complains of poor sexual satisfaction, what is your first reaction?
11. If the psycho-sexologist proposes NOT to implant the prosthesis in a patient, how do you usually deal with the situation?

20.11 Medical History Questions

20.11.1 For the Patient

1. How did you come to the hypothesis of a prosthetic implant? And what do you expect from this treatment?
2. What most did you miss in your previous sexual experience, using oral or injective drugs?
3. How did you experience those practices? Alone, in secret, sharing them with your partner?
4. Have you ever had extramarital relationships to try to overcome severe erectile dysfunction?
5. What do you mean by severe erectile function?
6. Who, apart from the specialists, did you talk to about your problem?
7. How many hours a day did you spend thinking about erectile dysfunction?
8. Have you ever looked for alternative solutions on the Internet? (e.g., drugs)
9. How did the andrologist surgeon choose to implant your prosthesis?
10. What struck you the most about the personality of the andrologist surgeon?
11. How influential was your partner's judgment in choosing to come here (to the clinic)?

20.11.2 For the Partner

1. What part do you think you yourself have played in getting your partner to resolve severe erectile dysfunction?
2. Have you ever felt defeated? With a great desire to leave everything behind?
3. Have you ever thought about ending your relationship with your partner?

4.	Is this the first time you have experienced a difficult sexuality with a partner?
5.	Have you ever suffered, even occasionally, from decreased desire, excitement disorder, or vagin ismus?
6.	If you were currently experiencing a personal sexual difficulty, how would you feel about seeing your partner so involved in resolving severe erectile dysfunction?
7.	Have you ever been afraid that your partner would no longer want to resolve erectile dysfunction?
8.	How much do you talk, as a couple, about your sexual desires and not only about the problems of intimacy?
9.	Who have you spoken to so far about your relationship?
10.	How do you think your life will change as a couple after the implantation?
11.	Do you think that your partner might want (once reassured by the prosthetic implant) to share sexuality with other partners?

References

1. Virag R et al (1981) Vascular impotence: a review of 92 cases with 54 surgeries. Vasc Surg 15:9–17
2. Gandaglia G et al (2014) A systemic review of the association between erectile dysfunction and cardiovascular disease. Eur Urol 65:968–978
3. Boddi V et al (2010) Priapus is happier with Venus with Bacchus. J Sex Med 7:2831–2841
4. Corona G et al (2005) Smoke psychobiological correlations in patients with erectile dysfunction. Int J Impot Res 17:527–534
5. Wang F et al (2013) Erectile dysfunction and fruit/vegetable consumption among diabetic Canadian men. Urology 82:1330–1335
6. Corona G et al (2013) The study IMMEDIATELY-DE: sexual dysfunction in patients with newly diagnosed type 2 diabetes. J Endocrinol Investig 36:864–868
7. Corona G et al (2014a) Sexual dysfunction at onset of diabetes 2: interaction between depression, cardiovascular and hormonal factors. J Sex Med 11:2065–2073
8. Corona G et al (2014b) Erectile dysfunction and obesity: an Italian perspective. Asian J Androl 16:581–591
9. Nelson CJ et al (2011) The association between erectile dysfunction and depressive symptoms. J Sex Med 8:560–566
10. Shabsigh R et al (1998) Increased incidence of depressive symptoms in men with erectile dysfunction. Urology 52:848–852
11. Huang SA et al (2013) Phosphodiesterase 5 (PDE5) in managing erectile dysfunction. PT 38:407–419
12. Shover LR et al (2002) Definition of sexual outcomes following treatment for localized prostate cancer. Cancer 95:1773–1785
13. Jiann BP et al (2013) The female sexual function is related to the erectile function of male partners? J Sex Med 10:420–429
14. Fisher WA et al (2006) Sexual experience of partners of men with erectile dysfunction: the female experience in front of the two life events and sexuality. J Sex Med 2(5):675–684
15. Trost LW et al (2013) Long-term outcomes of penile prosthesis for the treatment of erectile dysfunction. Expert Rev Med Devices 10(3):353–366

Bibliography

Levine LA, Becher E, Bella A et al (2016) Penile prosthesis surgery: current recommendations from the International Consultation on Sexual Medicine. J Sex Med 13(4):489–518. https://doi.org/10.1016/j.jsxm.2016.01.017. Epub 2016 Mar 25

Hakky TS, Wang R, Henry GD (2014) The evolution of the inflatable penile prosthetic device and surgical innovations with anatomical considerations. Curr Urol Rep 15(6):410

Trost L, Hellstrom W (2013) History, contemporary outcomes, and future of penile prostheses: a review of the literature. Sex Med Rev 1:150–163

Natali A, Olianas R, Fisch M (2008) Penile implantation in Europe: successes and complications with 253 implants in Italy and Germany. J Sex Med 5:1503–1512

Eid F, Wilson SK, Cleves M et al (2012) Coated implants and "no touch" surgical technique decreases risk of infection in inflatable penile prosthesis implantation to 0.46%. Urology 79:1310–1315

Bettocchi C, Palumbo F, Spilotros M et al (2010) Patient and partner satisfaction after AMS inflatable penile prosthesis implant. J Sex Med 7:304–309

Akin-Olugbade O, Parker M, Guhring P et al (2006) Determinants of patient satisfaction following penile prosthesis surgery. J Sex Med 3:743–748

21 A Clinical Experience: Two-Year Experience with Post-surgical Sexual Rehabilitation in Alto Adige

Armin Pycha and Emanuela Trenti

The Central Hospital of Bolzano is a referral hospital for the Trentino-Alto Adige Region and has a catchment area covering 270,000 people. Approximately 41,000 patients are admitted each year. With the exception of cardiac surgery, all surgical disciplines are represented. The hospital covers all common surgical procedures. In general surgery, thoracic surgery, and urology, new laparoscopic surgical techniques are also regularly performed.

The Department of Urology has 28 beds for ordinary admissions and 2 beds for day hospital admissions. The department is staffed by 11 doctors, 24 nurses, 5 technicians, and a nurse specialized in urodynamics. Annually, 1700 patients are admitted, and 18,000 outpatient services are provided. One operating room for open surgery and one for endourological surgery are available every day, while every year, 3500 surgical DRGs are performed in the urological department.

The scope of surgical activity encompasses all major ablative surgical interventions along with the related lower urinary tract surgical reconstruction techniques and radical prostatectomy.

Since the year 2000, approximately 60 cystoprostatectomies and 70 radical prostatectomies have been performed annually. In about half of these cases, retropubic access is used, with perineal access being used in the other half, depending on the surgical risk and the preference of the patient. Laparoscopic prostatectomy is not currently offered.

When in April 2000 the Urology Department was taken over by the new director, there was no expert staff available, meaning that a completely new surgical team had to be trained. It is of course clear that the surgical aspect of the operation has to be placed in the foreground: employees have to be trained, but at the same time, the learning curve has to be kept as high as possible. This means offering a high-quality service without compromising the rate of complications and at the same time obtaining a more precise and higher level of training for employees. For this reason, a quality control system was introduced in order to provide data that can be compared with the reference centers: thus far, each patient has been entered in a database, where all events and tests are recorded, both oncological and non-oncological.

E. V. Longhi et al., *Psychosexual Counseling in Andrological Surgery*,
https://doi.org/10.1007/978-3-319-99646-2_21

It is therefore understandable that we can find very little time for the social aspect related to these oncological diseases. There are two reasons for this:

- During the primary surgical training, little value is given to this aspect. There was no structured training in patient interviews on topics such as impotence, incontinence, sexual behavior, and changes in interpersonal relationships: what you cannot do and what you do not like doing are considered less important.
- Organizational and technical aspects remain in the foreground in order to train nurses and doctors and to become familiar with both new operating techniques and postoperative care.

Both the merits and the shortcomings of the supervisor are automatically transmitted to the personnel. It soon became clear that, in this respect, there was a pressing need for improvement. Initially, an attempt was made to find a remedy within the department.

Every patient who had to undergo a cystectomy or a prostatectomy was, following a general explanation of the surgical procedure, invited to a second or third interview along with their partner, during which the social and sexual aspects were also addressed. This led to a marked improvement in patient treatment but often also to a situation of considerable overload for the doctor. Furthermore, the approach to sexual relations and sexual problems could not be adequately developed.

The need for more specialized help, as much for the good of the patients as for the doctors, became clear. The internal psychological service of the hospital refused the request for help on two grounds: on the one hand, they would not have had enough resources to guarantee this type of continuous care; on the other, all these issues should already have been implicit in the psycho-oncological care.

During a congress, I met Dr. Elena Vittoria Longhi, an expert in sexual therapy, who declared herself willing to fill this gap. Under an agreement with the Health Unit of Bolzano and third-party financing, her collaboration was guaranteed for 2 years.

From September 2002, the care of patients who underwent a major ablative intervention followed this protocol:

- First interview on the communication of the diagnosis
- Second interview when the type of treatment was decided
- Third interview, with the partner
- Introduction to the psychosexologist
- Introduction to stoma therapists
- Surgical intervention
- Removal of the bladder catheter
- Visit by stoma therapists with an individually agreed checkup
- Discharge
- First inspection visit 7–10 days after discharge
- Uro-oncological follow-up with a follow-up visit at 3-monthly intervals
- Androcheck at regular intervals

What had changed then with the introduction of therapeutic sexual treatment? The presence of the psychosexologist, Doctor Elena Vittoria Longhi, was initially limited to two visits a month, later increased to four. On the days of her presence, after the morning handover, a briefing was held at 8.15 a.m. attended by the doctors, nurses, stoma therapists, the urodynamic nurse, and the psychosexologist. The patient was introduced by a colleague who provided all relevant information and tried to carry out a social evaluation. Stoma therapists provided continence data, while the Androcheck specialist contributed data regarding sexual interest. In this way, the psychosexologist received the first impression of the patient. The novelty here was that the different disciplines were all sitting together at the same table and exchanging information about the same person. New facets, impressions, data, and details that were previously unknown were now accessible to everyone. The patient was treated by, in the true sense of the word, a team.

In the evening, de-briefing took place: Doctor Longhi gave a response regarding the initial measures, the social and psychological aspects, and information about any shortcomings in the care so that these could be remedied immediately. What became immediately clear was the fact that in this way, everyone knew the patient much more fully. It was also particularly instructive that 74% of the patients treated by the psychotherapist had already had relationship problems before the operation: thus the disease became a new opportunity for the patient himself and for the couple. It was often suggested that a psychiatrist or neurologist should be consulted. The service network became more fine-tuned and offered a more specific service ad personam. And each of us benefitted: the patient through better care and us through greater knowledge and greater awareness of our work.

What are the concrete advantages that we urologists gained from this experience?

- New team spirit
- A more intimate personal and interdisciplinary understanding of the patient within the sphere of the team
- An understanding of new perspectives in the evaluation of the sick person (one learns to look back, to record the problem, because one knows that as a therapist, one is not left alone)
- Extension of the medical repertoire
- Confidence in the approach to the patient and his problems
- Feedback
- Increased sense of success

What benefits did the patient receive?

- Optimal multidisciplinary treatment
- The feeling of not being left alone
- Appropriate rehabilitation in the social, sexual, and medical spheres

Was our model successful?

This question must undoubtedly be answered with a yes. This approach to treatment was so successful that it was bound for failure. At first, the patients were skeptical. Very often we heard the phrase: "But Doctor, that's not important to me." So we agreed with the patient to make at least one first visit to get to know the therapist. The patient would then have been free to pass up on the offer, had it not been to his liking. In 2 years, only one patient refused to continue treatment after the first visit, deeming it unnecessary.

The success of the treatment became known so quickly by word of mouth among patients that it was initially extended to nephrectomized patients. We then received a request from stoma therapists to offer this type of care to patients with ileocolostomy as well. We were presented with a number of requests. The next step was therefore to include these conditions in our project. The agreed number of hours was no longer adequate, and the presence of the psychosexologist had to cover a total of four specialties.

Through various self-help groups, our project was also made known in other cities in Alto Adige, and a large number of patients requested the opportunity to receive this type of treatment. Programs had already been planned for the entire province, including at the level of the Department of Health, when there was a surprising turn of events.

The psychologists of the hospital's internal service presented a report stating that they would learn everything they needed, that they would be able to offer this form of assistance, and that a renewal of the agreement would no longer be necessary. It would therefore have been possible to use the money elsewhere. Given the increasingly limited financial resources, this proposal was well received by the administration of the hospital, which thus did not renew the agreement.

Since then, there has been no therapeutic sexual assistance in public hospitals in Alto Adige. Patients obviously receive andrological assistance, but this concerns the physiology of the erection, its pathophysiology after iatrogenic damage, and the consequent medical treatment. All the psychological aspects of the relationship with the partner, and the concomitant change in sexuality, are left unattended. What is seen as essential and standard in the field of oncology, namely, psychological help in returning to life, is not considered necessary in the field of sexuality. The sexual sphere, which is still taboo in social life, is therefore still excluded. It is surprising that self-help groups do not assert their rights in the same way as they had successfully done before.

In the end, it has to be said that this "sexual rehabilitation" project was too successful not to arouse envy. It is precisely this envy, among psychologists though not among doctors, that led to our failure. It is regrettable but true that one of the richest provinces in Italy is not able to offer help in this area to its patients, who are the ones who suffer the consequences. Here there was a good approach, but we were tripped up by something human, maybe something all too human.

FSC
www.fsc.org
MIX
Papier aus verantwortungsvollen Quellen
Paper from responsible sources
FSC® C105338

If you have any concerns about our products,
you can contact us on
ProductSafety@springernature.com

In case Publisher is established outside the EU,
the EU authorized representative is:
Springer Nature Customer Service Center GmbH
Europaplatz 3, 69115 Heidelberg, Germany

Printed by Libri Plureos GmbH
in Hamburg, Germany